# Essentials of
# Traumatic Injuries
# to the Teeth

# J.O. Andreasen and F.M. Andreasen

# Essentials of Traumatic Injuries to the Teeth

Department of Oral Medicine and Oral Surgery,
University Hospital (Rigshospitalet), Copenhagen, Denmark

Departments of Pediatric Dentistry and
Oral and Maxillofacial Surgery,
Royal Dental College, Copenhagen, Denmark

Munksgaard

Essentials of Traumatic Injuries to the Teeth
1st edition, 2nd printing 1991
Copyright © 1990 J.O.Andreasen, F.M.Andreasen and
Munksgaard, Copenhagen
All rights reserved

Medical illustrations by HDC design, Henning Dalhoff Christiansen
Cover and lay-out by Lars Thorsen
Typesetting by P.J.Schmidt, Vojens
Reproduction by High Tech Repro A/S, Copenhagen
Printed in Denmark by Laursen A/S, Tønder

ISBN 87-16-10414-5

# Contents

# Foreword

One feature common to all patients presenting with acute dental trauma is the fact that they come to us unexpectedly. There is no spot in our appointment books designated "*Trauma.*" They just come. It can be in the midst of a busy day, where others are waiting patiently or impatiently for treatment; or in the middle of the night.

The purpose of this atlas is to provide the clinician, whether in a dental practice or emergency service of a hospital, with a readily accessible guide to initial treatment of acute dental trauma. In that regard, in order to facilitate initial examination and record-keeping, Appendix 1 provides a standardized emergency chart that can be used. Moreover, Appendix 2 provides a standardized clinical examination form for acute and follow-up examinations. Appendix 3 summarizes the clinical and radiographic characteristics of each luxation category. It is suggested that these or similar forms be duplicated and completed as an integral part of the trauma patient's record.

In the case of some trauma entities, such as concussion, subluxation and some injuries to the primary dentition, observation "therapy" is the only treatment needed. In other situations, repositioning and splinting procedures characterize treatment. Techniques for the reduction of tooth dislocations include immediate repositioning or repositioning using an orthodontic or surgical approach. The decision of which procedure to employ will be discussed. Finally Appendix 4 is aimed at assisting in determining when the patient should be seen in order to detect changes in the follow-up period which might necessitate interceptive therapy.

It is the authors' hope that *Essentials of Traumatic Injuries to the Teeth* will serve to aid the dental clinician in providing optimal care to the acutely traumatized patient, thereby reducing the stress and anxiety of the first treatment episode - for both the patient and the clinician.

Those readers who are interested in an in-depth discussion of the biological impact of the various trauma entities upon the pulp and periodontium, the pathogenesis of the various healing complications and long-term effects and treatment of oral trauma are referred to the textbook, *Traumatic Injuries to the Teeth*.

Finally, the authors would like to express their gratitude to Drs. Miomir Cvek and Barbro Malmgren, Department of Pedodontics at the Eastman Dental Institute, Stockholm, Sweden, for their valuable contributions to the chapters on crown and crown-root fractures. We also thank the staff of the Department of Oral Medicine and Oral Surgery, University Hospital, Copenhagen and the Departments of Pediatric Dentistry and Oral and Maxillofacial Surgery, Royal Dental College, Copenhagen.

*Jens O. Andreasen*                    *Frances M. Andreasen*

*Copenhagen, 1990*

# Examination of the traumatized patient

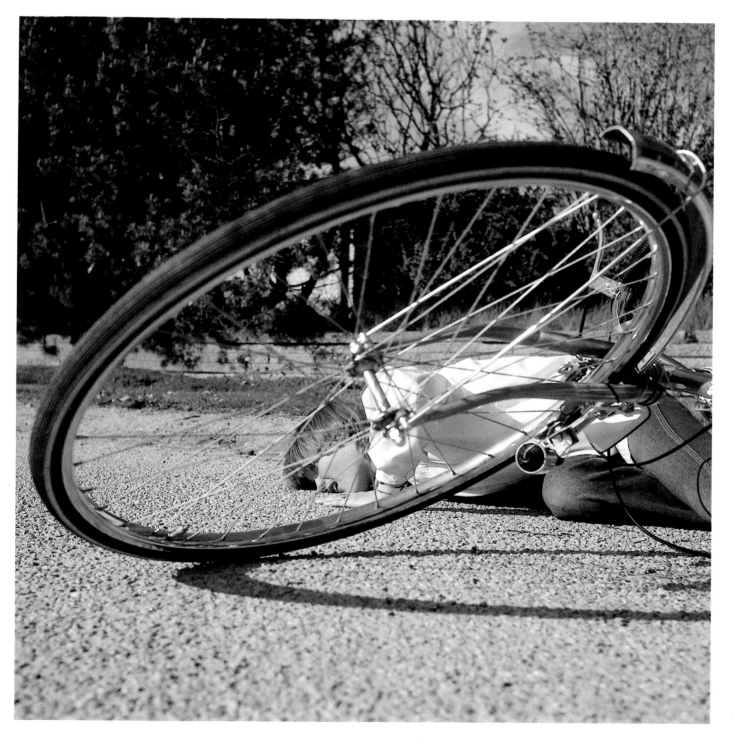

EXAMINATION OF THE TRAUMATIZED PATIENT

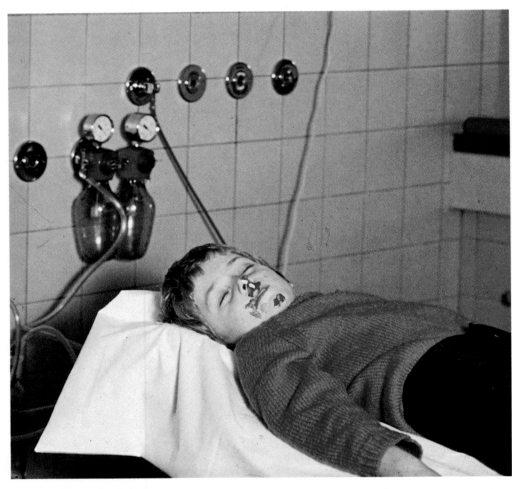

Fig. 1.1. Examination of the injured patient

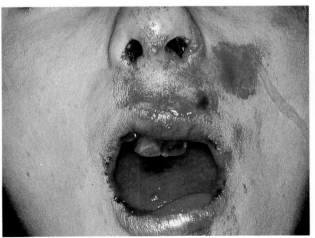
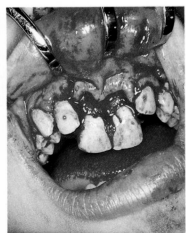

CHAPTER 1

# Examination of the traumatized patient

In order to arrive at a quick and correct diagnosis of the probable extent of injury to the pulp, periodontium and associated structures, a systematic examination of the traumatized patient is essential and will be demonstrated in the following.

When the patient is received for treatment of an acute trauma, the oral region is usually heavily contaminated (Fig. 1.1). The first step in the examination procedure, therefore, is to wash the patient's face. In case of soft tissue wounds, a mild detergent should be used (see later). While this is being done, it is possible to get an initial impression of the extent of injury. Thereafter, a series of questions must be asked to aid in diagnosis and treatment planning.

These questions include:

**How did the injury occur?** The answer will indicate the location of possible injury zones (e.g. crown-root fractures in the premolar and molar region after impacts under the chin) (Fig. 1.2).

**Where did the injury occur?** While there might be legal implications in the answer to this question, this will also indicate the possibility of contamination of wounds.

**When did the injury occur?** The answer will imply a time factor, which could influence the choice of treatment. This time factor becomes critical in the case of avulsed or displaced teeth.

Fig. 1.2. **Trauma direction**
The direction of impact determines the pattern of injury. A blow to the chin has resulted in multiple cusp fractures in the premolar and molar regions.

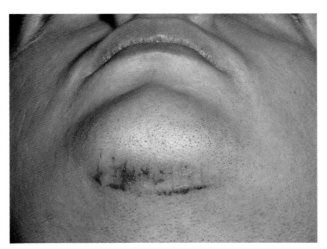
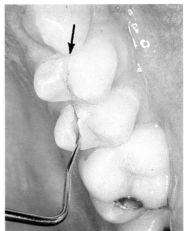

11

Finally any inconsistency between the appearance of the wounds on a child and the history supplied should raise the suspicion of the battered child syndrome. In this case, the patient should also be examined by a pediatrician.

**Was there a period of unconsciousness? If so, for how long? Is there headache? amnesia? nausea? vomiting?** These are all signs of brain concussion and require medical attention. However, this does not contraindicate immediate treatment of the dental injury. Early treatment will in most cases improve later prognosis.

**Has there been previous injury to the teeth?** Answers to this question may explain radiographic findings, such as pulp canal obliteration and incomplete root formation in a dentition with otherwise completed root development (Figs. 1.3 and 1.4).

**Is there any disturbance in the bite?** An affirmative answer can imply one of the following conditions: tooth luxation, alveolar fracture, jaw fracture or luxation or fracture of the temporomandibular joint.

**Is there any reaction in the teeth to cold and/or heat?** A positive finding indicates exposure of dentin and therefore need for dentinal coverage.

Finally, a short **medical history** should reveal possible allergies, blood diseases and other information which could influence treatment.

## The clinical examination

The clinical examination should first include examination of soft tissue wounds. If present, the penetrating nature of these should be determined, with emphasis on the possible presence of foreign bodies embedded within these wounds. Thereafter, the hard dental tissues are examined for the presence of infractions and fractures. The diagnosis of *infractions* is facilitated by directing the light beam parallel to the labial surface of the injured tooth (Fig. 1.5).

**Fig. 1.3. Previous injury, primary dentition**
This 4-year-old girl has suffered subluxation of her right central incisor. At the age of 1 year there was an injury affecting both central incisors resulting in pulp necrosis of the right central incisor and pulp canal obliteration of the left incisor.

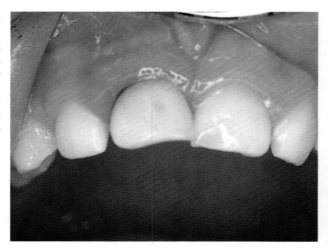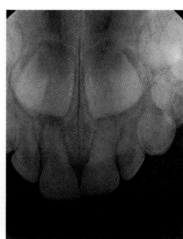

CHAPTER 1

In the case of *crown fractures* all possible pulp exposures should be detected and their size noted, as well as the vascularity of the pulp (whether there is fresh hemorrhage, cyanosis or ischemia). Detection of pinpoint perforations is facilitated by thorough cleansing of the fracture surface.

**Mobility testing** should determine the extent of loosening, especially in axial direction of individual teeth (an indication of a severed vascular supply) and mobility of groups of teeth (an indication of fracture of the alveolar process).

**Percussion testing**, with a finger in small children or the handle of a metal instrument, has two functions. Tenderness to percussion in an axial direction (i.e. from the incisal edge) will indicate damage to the periodontal ligament. Percussion of the labial surface will yield either a high or low percussion tone. A high, metallic percussion tone is an indication that the injured tooth is locked into bone (as in lateral luxation or intrusion). At the follow-up periods, this tone indicates ankylosis. This finding can be confirmed if a finger is placed on the oral surface of the tooth to be tested. It is possible to feel the tapping of the instrument in a tooth with a normal PDL. In the case of intrusion, lateral luxation or ankylosis, percussion cannot be felt through the tooth tested.

**Electrometric sensibility testing** should be carried out if at all possible, as it gives important information about the neurovas-

Fig. 1.4. **Previous injury, permanent dentition**
The patient has just suffered enamel fractures of the two central incisors. However, a dental injury 4 years earlier has resulted in pulp necrosis of both central incisors and pulp canal obliteration and arrested root formation of the left lateral incisor.

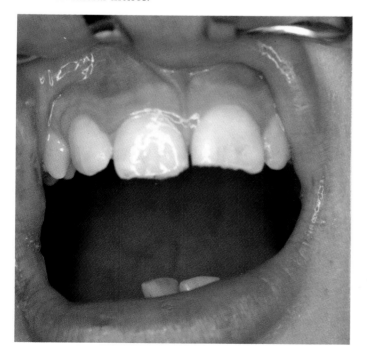
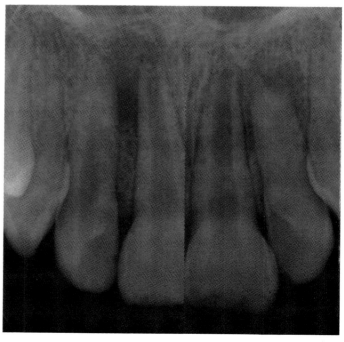

13

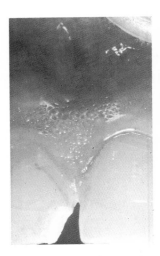
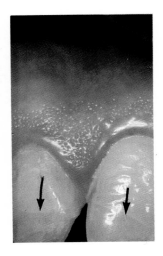

Fig. 1.5. **Diagnosing infractions**
When the light beam is directed parallel to the labial surface infractions become very prominent.

cular supply to the involved teeth. The most reliable response is obtained when the electrode is placed upon the incisal edge or the most incisal aspect of enamel in the case of crown fractures. It should be noted that young teeth with incomplete root formation do not respond consistently to sensibility testing; but the response at the time of injury provides a baseline value for comparison at later follow-up examinations. Finally, sensibility testing in the primary dentition may yield inconclusive information due to lack of patient cooperation.

In Appendix 1, an example of the emergency records used at the University Hospital dental department in Copenhagen is presented (see pages 155 to 158).

Appendix 2 provides a sample of the clinical examination form used at the time of injury and at follow-up examinations (see page 159).

Fig. 1.6. **Penetrating lip lesion**
Two parallel lesions, either in the mucosa and skin or mucosa only, are an indication that teeth have penetrated tissue and that tooth fragments and other foreign bodies can be expected deep within the wound. A radiographic film is placed between the lips and the dental arch. The exposure time is 25% of the normal.

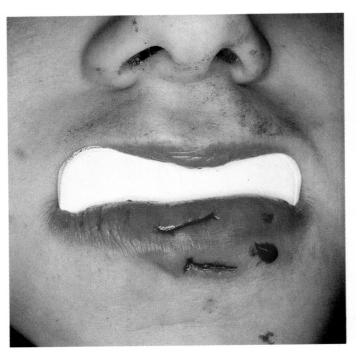
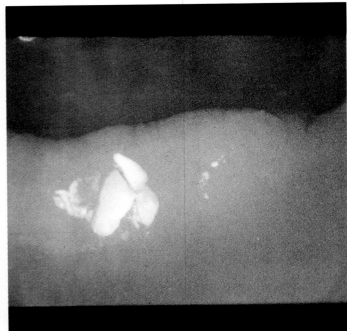

14

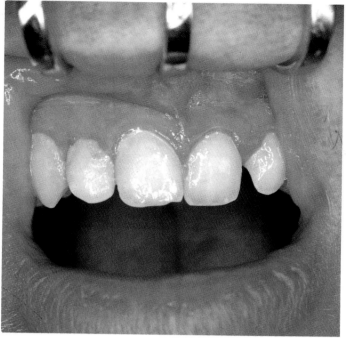
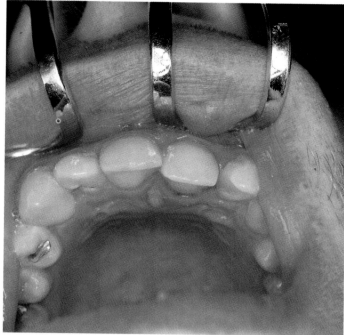

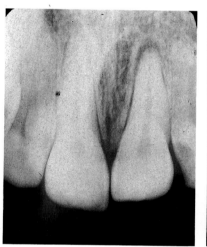
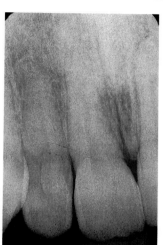
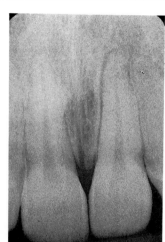
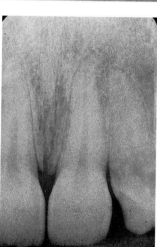

**Fig. 1.7. Complete radiographic and photographic examination of an anterior trauma**
Note how the injuries appear different on different exposures. Photographic registration of the trauma allows exact measurement of tooth displacement at a later date as well as complete documentation of the extent of injury. This injury consisted of lateral luxation of the left central incisor. Note how the occlusal exposure is superior in showing the lateral displacement.

## The radiographic examination

The clinical examination should now have determined the area of injury; that is the area to be examined radiographically. In the presence of a *penetrating lip lesion*, a soft tissue radiograph is indicated in order to locate eventual foreign bodies. It should be noted that the orbicularis oris muscles close tightly around foreign bodies in the lip, making them impossible to palpate; they can only be identified radiographically. This is accomplished by placing a dental film between the lips and the dental arch and using 25% of the normal exposure time (Fig. 1.6).

An occlusal exposure (using a size 2 film) of the traumatized anterior region gives an excellent view of most *lateral luxations, apical and mid-root root fractures* and *alveolar fractures* (Fig. 1.7)  **15**

The standard periapical bisecting angle exposure of each traumatized tooth (using a size 1 film) gives information about *cervical root fractures* as well as other tooth displacements. Thus, a radiographic examination comprising 1 occlusal exposure and 3 periapical bisecting angle exposures of the traumatized region will provide maximum information in determining the extent of trauma.

With the combined information from the clinical and radiographic examinations, diagnosis and treatment planning can then be carried out.

Finally, photographic registration of the trauma is recommended, as it offers an exact documentation of the extent of injury which can be used in later treatment planning, legal claims, or for clinical research.

In the following the examination, features of a typical trauma case resulting from a fall from a bicycle are shown (Fig. 1.8).

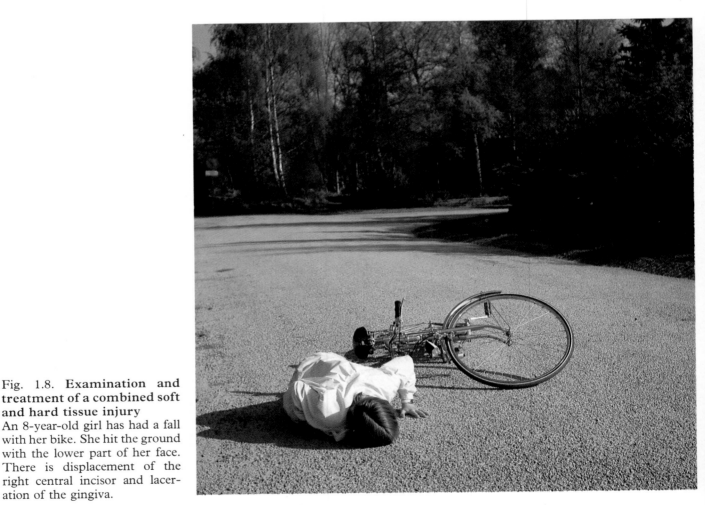

**Fig. 1.8. Examination and treatment of a combined soft and hard tissue injury**
An 8-year-old girl has had a fall with her bike. She hit the ground with the lower part of her face. There is displacement of the right central incisor and laceration of the gingiva.

**Extra- and intraoral lesions**
The lips show extensive abrasions with asphalt tattoos.

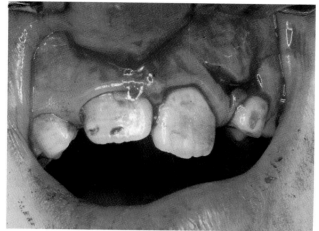 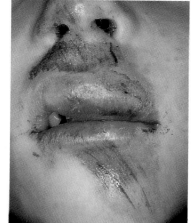

**Cleaning the patient**
The patient's face is washed with a mild wound detergent and the oral cavity rinsed with a water spray.

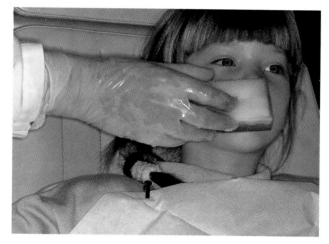 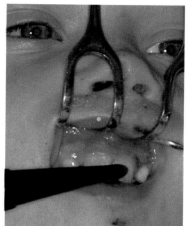

**Percussion test**
This test is first carried out on non-traumatized teeth so that the patient fully understands the proper reaction to this test. In this case both horizontal and vertical percussion gave no sensitivity reaction; and the percussion tone was high and metallic, indicating that the displaced tooth was forced into the alveolus.

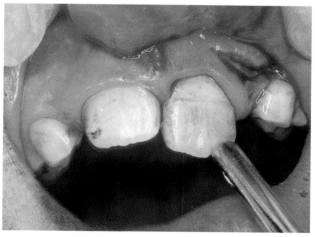 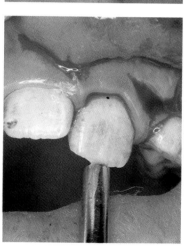

**Mobility and sensibility testing**
Mobility is tested in vertical as well as in horizontal direction. In this case the tooth was immobile. Sensibility testing should always be carried out on the incisal edge in order to get maximum stimulation of the pulp. In this case there was no response to pulp testing.

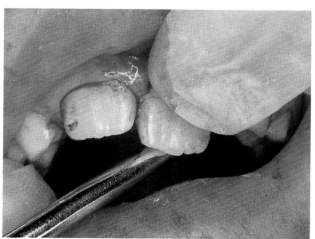 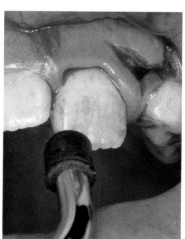

EXAMINATION OF THE TRAUMATIZED PATIENT

### Radiographic examination

A complete examination is made including an occlusal exposure and three bisecting angle radiographs. Note how the occlusal exposure (arrow) is optimal for showing the apical displacement.

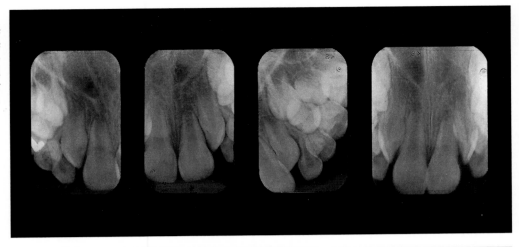

### Repositioning and splinting

The laterally luxated incisor is repositioned and splinted and the gingival laceration sutured.

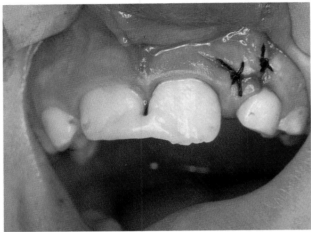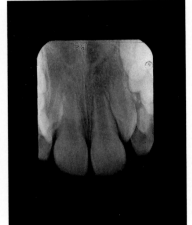

### Rinsing the skin wounds

In order to adequately cleanse the abrasions, a topical anesthetic is necessary. In this case a lidocain spray was used. Note that the nostrils are compressed during the spraying procedure in order to reduce discomfort caused by spray entering the nose.

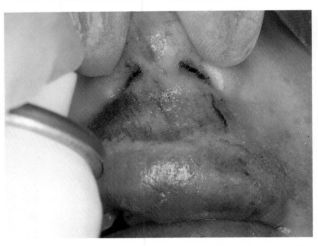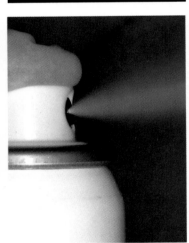

### Washing the wounds

The lips are washed with surgical sponges or gauze sponges soaked in a wound detergent.

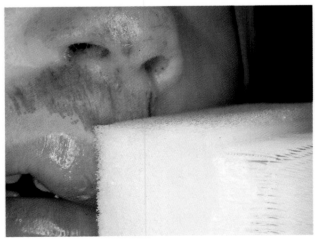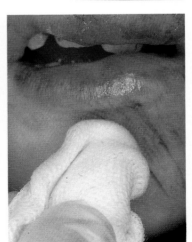

18

**Removing asphalt particles**
The impacted foreign bodies cannot be adequately removed by scrubbing or washing, but should be removed with a small excavator or a surgical blade kept perpendicular to the direction of the abrasions.

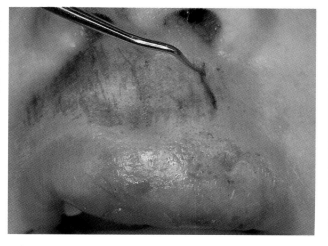
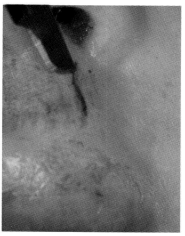

**Follow-up**
Two weeks after injury, the soft tissue wounds have healed without scarring and the injured tooth is in normal position.

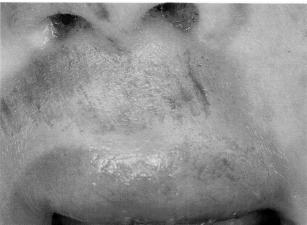
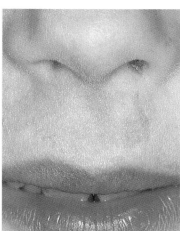

## Essentials
- Obtain standardized data from the patient.
- Clean the traumatized region.
- History: When, where and how did the injury occur?
- Unconsciousness? amnesia? headache? nausea? vomiting?
- Disturbance in the bite?
- Reaction to cold or heat?
- Previous dental injury?
- Any allergies or serious illness?

**Clinical examination**
- Soft tissue.
- Hard tissues (enamel fracture, dentin or pulp exposures)?
- Abnormal mobility, tooth displacement.
- Tenderness to percussion, percussion (ankylosis) tone.
- Electrometric pulpal sensibility.

**Radiographic examination**
- Soft tissues.
- Occlusal radiographic exposure of the anterior region.
- Periapical bisecting angle exposure of each traumatized tooth.

**Final diagnosis and treatment planning**

# CHAPTER 2

# Crown fractures

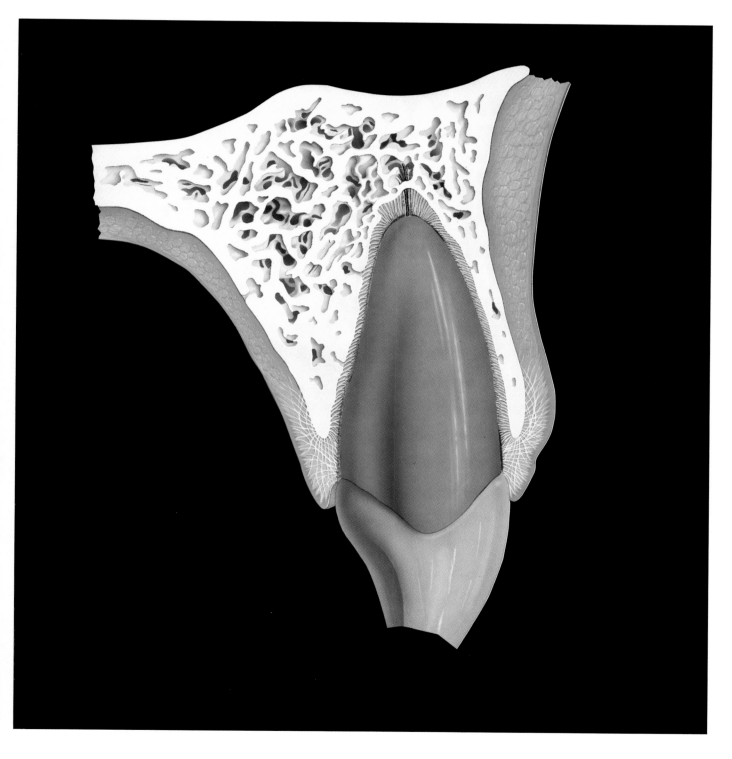

21

Fig. 2.1. A frontal impact results in a crown fracture

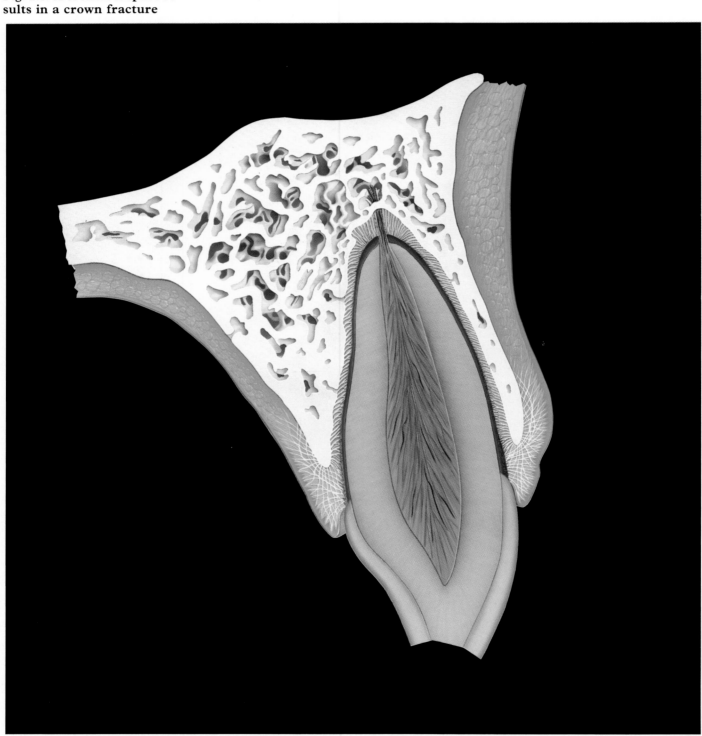

# Pattern of injury and diagnosis

Crown fractures comprise the most frequent injuries in the permanent dentition. Apart from the loss of hard tissue, this injury can represent a hazard to the pulp. The usual cause of a crown fracture is a frontal impact, the energy of which exceeds the shear strength of enamel and dentin (Fig. 2.1). The tooth is thereby fractured in a horizontal pattern, following the course of the enamel rods. If the impact is from another direction, other lines of fracture may be seen. Pulpal status following crown fracture depends upon various factors: whether there is a concomitant luxation injury and the stage of root development, whether dentin has been exposed and, if so, the time interval from injury until dentinal coverage (as well as the type of dentinal coverage).

The closeness of the fracture to the pulp and the risk of bacteria or bacterial toxins penetrating dentin into the pulp are the primary sources of pulpal complications after crown fracture. In the

**Fig. 2.2. Treatment of enamel fracture**
Symmetry is reestablished by selective grinding of the injured and adjacent incisor.

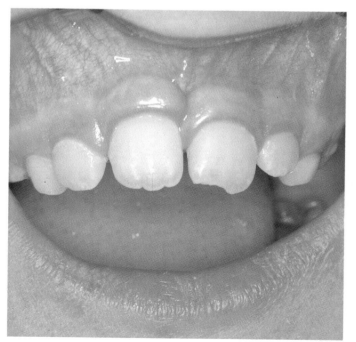
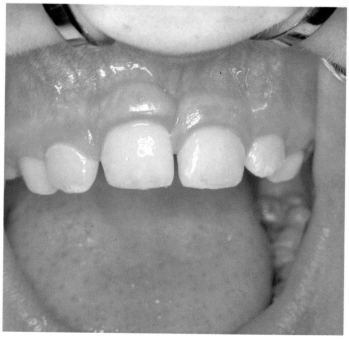

23

case of untreated, uncomplicated crown fractures, bacterial plaque will accumulate on the exposed dentin, later to invade dentinal tubules. The rate of invasion and its significance for pulpal status is not known.

In case of a pulp exposure, the following events take place. Soon after injury, the exposed pulp is covered with a layer of fibrin. A zone of acute inflammation is seen immediately subjacent to the exposure site. After 2 days, proliferative changes take place, whereby the pulp ultimately protrudes through the exposure. A significant finding is that the inflammatory zone is still confined to the most superficial 1-2 mm of the pulp even 1 week after injury. In case of an associated luxation injury, these events may be modified by total ischemia and autolysis of the pulp.

## Treatment

In some cases of *enamel fractures*, selective grinding of the incisal edge is sufficient. In other cases, restoration with composite and the acid-etch technique is indicated. The extent and location of the fracture dictates the choice of treatment (Fig. 2.2).

On the other hand, *fractures of enamel and dentin* always require restoration in order to seal dentinal tubules and to restore esthe-

Fig. 2.3. Treatment of an uncomplicated crown fracture with composite resin and the acid-etch technique

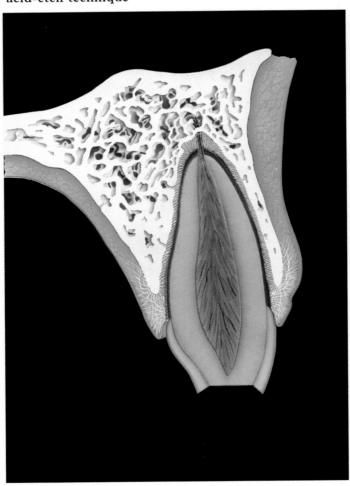
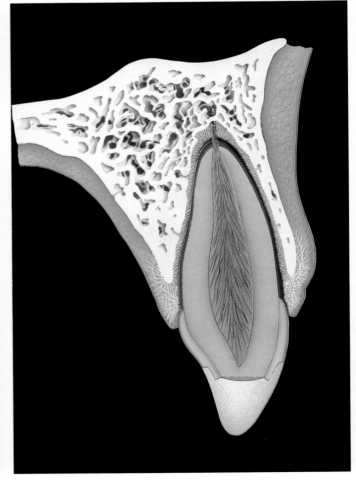

24

tics. Restoration of esthetics can be achieved by composite resin build-up (Figs. 2.3 and 2.4), reattachment of the crown fragment using a dentin bonding agent, or by full crown restoration.

At the time of injury, various factors can influence the choice of treatment as well as whether or not immediate definitive treatment can be performed. In many situations, a temporary restoration may be indicated. These include pulpal involvement, concomitant luxation injuries and lack of patient cooperation. Temporary restoration can be in the form of a pre-formed stainless steel or resin crown or temporary build-up using a temporary crown and bridge material. If pre-formed crowns are to be cemented in place, it should be remembered that, in the case of concomitant luxation injuries, the periodontal ligament has been ruptured. In these cases, care must be taken to avoid forcing the temporary luting agent into the injured periodontal ligament space.

With respect to maintaining pulpal vitality, successful restoration of enamel-dentin crown fractures requires a hermetic seal of exposed dentinal tubules. This can be achieved by using glass ionomer cement, hard setting calcium hydroxide paste or a dentin bonding agent (see later). While zinc oxide-eugenol cement has been found to be one of the best agents for producing a hermetic

**Fig. 2.4. Treatment of uncomplicated crown fracture with composite resin and acid-etch technique**
Uncomplicated crown fracture in a 19-year-old girl.

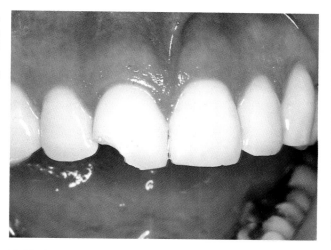
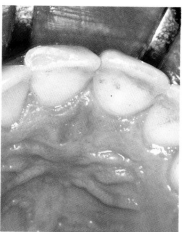

**Shade selection**
Shade selection should be made *after* polishing with pure pumice and water and *before* application of the rubber dam, as the dehydrated enamel will change color.

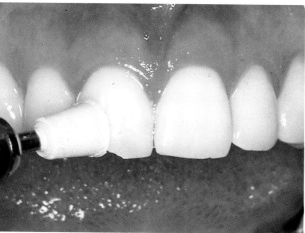
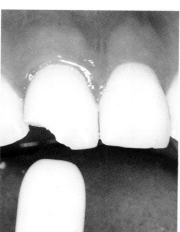

25

antibacterial seal, it is not recommended in situations where a composite resin restoration is to be placed, as the eugenol component will interfere with polymerization.

## Composite resin build-up (Fig. 2.4)

### Preparation

Preparation of teeth for composite build-up has long been a subject of debate. It has been found that a *chamfer margin* (in contrast to a bevel) yields the best final result due to ease of finishing and the greater bulk of material at the final margin. The best restorative result is achieved if a rubber dam is used.

### Dentinal coverage

Prior to acid etching and final restoration, dentinal coverage is necessary to protect pulpal vitality. This can be in the form of hard setting calcium hydroxide paste, glass ionomer cement or a dentin bonding agent (see later).

### Acid etching

In order to ensure a tight seal against microleakage following restoration, adequate acid etching is required. That is, 30 seconds' etch followed by rinsing of the etched enamel surface with a

**Application of a rubber dam**
A rubber dam is applied. Adjacent teeth should be included.

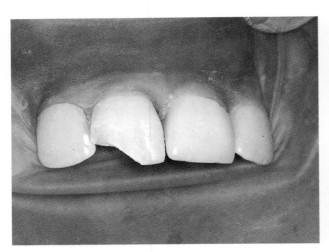
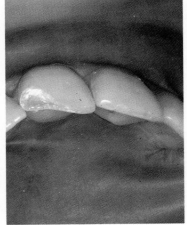

**Chamfer preparation**
A chamfer preparation is made labially and lingually, extending 2 mm from the fracture surface.

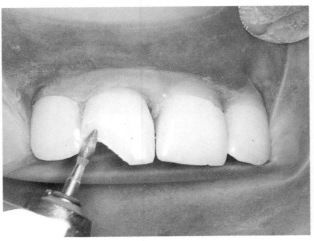
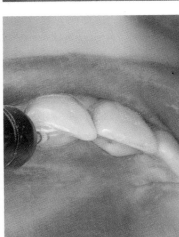

**Covering exposed dentin**
Exposed dentin is covered with a hard-setting calcium hydroxide cement.

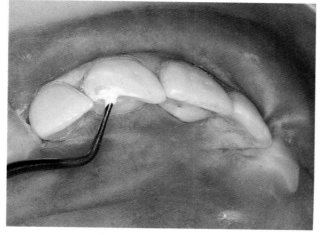
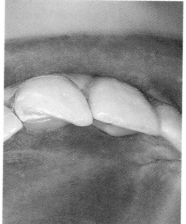

**Etching enamel**
The enamel is etched and a temporary crown form adapted.

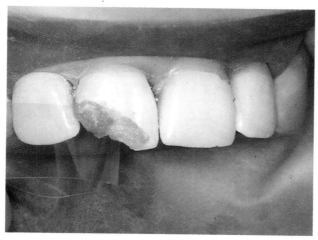
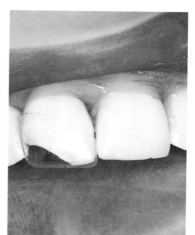

**Polymerization of composite**
After curing, the surface anatomy is defined with a finishing diamond, whereas the general polishing is made with discs.

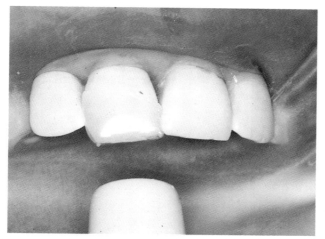
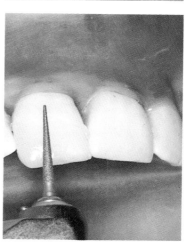

**Finished restoration**
Clinical and radiographic appearance of the restoration.

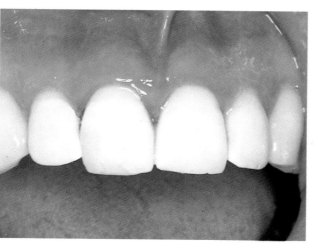
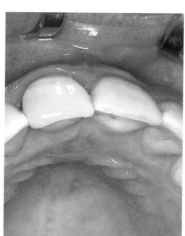

27

copious flow of water for 20 seconds in order to remove all traces of etchant. Thereafter air drying to yield the characteristic mat enamel surface.

### Choice of composite material

Light-cured resins have been found to possess the best color stability when compared with two-component self-cured resins. Crown fractures can be restored either using a layer build-up technique or by the use of standardized crown forms which are filled with the restorative material to be used. The choice of either technique is a personal one. However, it should be noted that light from the polymerizing lamp can only penetrate 2.0 mm and that in larger restorations adequate polymerization requires greater light exposure to achieve optimal material properties.

## Reattachment of the crown fragment (Fig. 2.6)

This form of treatment has been shown to yield good esthetic results in that original tooth anatomy is restored with a material that abrades at a rate identical to that of the adjacent tooth substance and at the same time permits continual monitoring of pulpal status through the fragment (Fig. 2.5).

### Clinical procedure (Fig. 2.5)

The enamel-dentin fragment can either be brought to the dental clinic at the time of injury or can be recovered later. All fragments should be stored in either physiologic saline or tap water until bonding to prevent discoloration and/or infractions due to dehydration.

In the case of *small uncomplicated fractures*, where there is a good distance from the fracture surface to the pulp, and no concomitant luxation injury, bonding can be performed immediately. However, following *profound uncomplicated fractures* (where the red of the pulp can be seen through dentin), and concomitant luxation *complicated fractures*, a period of temporary restoration must be included in the treatment schedule.

### Temporization

In *uncomplicated fractures*, the exposed fracture surface (enamel and dentin) is disinfected and then covered with hard-setting calcium hydroxide cement (e.g. Dycal®, Life®).

In *complicated fractures*, pure calcium hydroxide (e.g. Calasept®) is placed over the perforation. The enamel and dentin of the fracture surface are then covered with hard-setting calcium hydroxide. In both cases, the teeth are temporarily restored (4 wk for uncomplicated fractures; 3 months for complicated fractures) until bonding.

In the case of *concomitant luxation injuries*, the fixation period is the same as for the given trauma entity. However, for concomitant concussion or subluxation temporization of approximately 2 wk is recommended. The temporary restoration should stabilize the fractured tooth in order to avoid migration of the injured incisor or its antagonists. If preformed crowns are used, eugenol-containing cements should be avoided as eugenol can penetrate dentin and prevent optimal bonding.

### Bonding of crown fractures

The bonding procedure for an uncomplicated crown fracture is illustrated in Fig. 2.6.

In the case of a complicated fracture, pulpal considerations are discussed later. Bonding is carried out when there is hard tissue closure of the perforation, i.e. approximately 3 months after injury. At that time, the temporary restoration is removed and the fracture site examined. An intact hard tissue barrier should be present at the site of exposure. There should also be normal sensibility to pulp testing.

All soft tissue remnants from the exposure site are removed. The fracture surface is disinfected and the barrier covered with a calcium hydroxide dressing (e.g. Dycal® or Life®). Pulpal remnants in the crown fragment are removed with a round bur.

Fig. 2.5. Reattachment of crown fragment using a dentin bonding agent

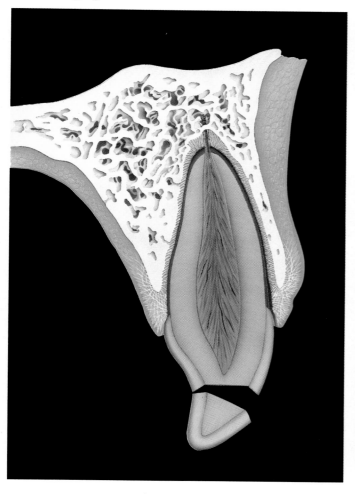
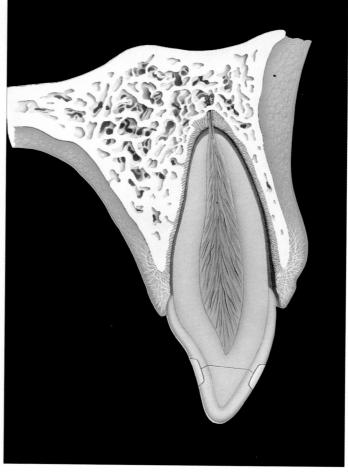

**Fig. 2.6. Treatment of an uncomplicated crown fracture by reattaching the crown fragment with a dentin bonding agent and reinforcement of the bonding site with composite resin and the acid-etch technique**

This 10-year-old boy has fractured his central incisor after a fall from his skateboard. The fracture is very close to the mesial pulp horn.

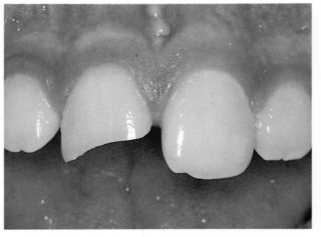
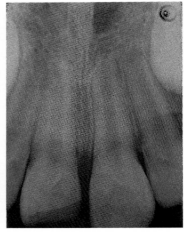

**Testing pulpal sensibility**
Pulpal response to sensibility testing is normal. The radiographic examination shows no displacement or root fracture.

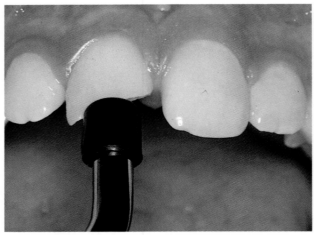
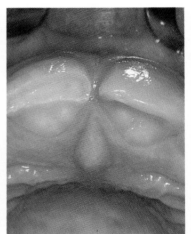

**Testing the fit of the fragment**
The fragment fits exactly. The enamel surface is intact, with no apparent defect at the enamel margins.

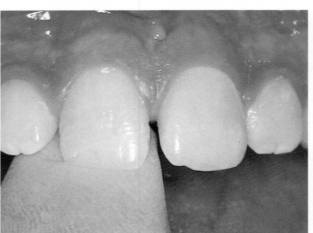
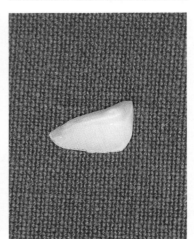

**Temporary dentin coverage with calcium hydroxide**
Due to the close proximity of the fracture surface to the pulp, a temporary calcium hydroxide dressing is placed over the entire fracture surface, including enamel, prior to placement of the temporary restoration.

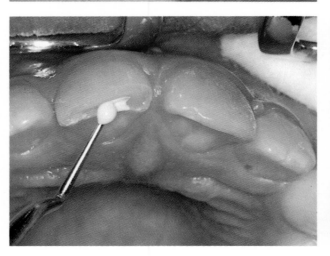
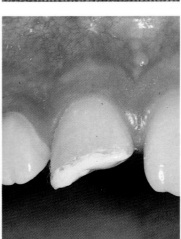

### Etching the enamel
A 2-mm wide zone of enamel around the fracture surface is etched.

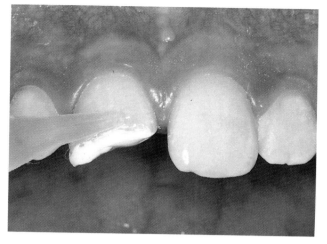 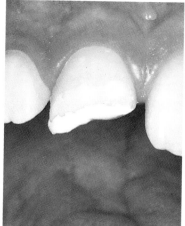

### Covering the fracture surface
The tooth is temporarily restored with a temporary crown and bridge material. To provide greater stability, the restoration may be extended to adjacent teeth.

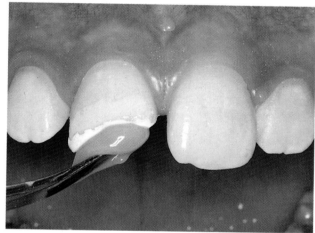 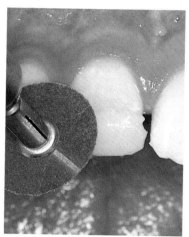

### Storage of the crown fragment
The tooth is stored in physiologic saline for 1 month. The patient is given the fragment and is instructed to change the solution once a week to reduce contamination.

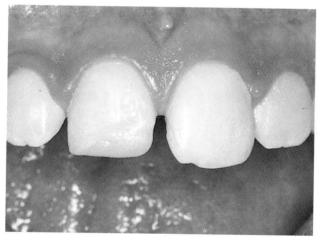 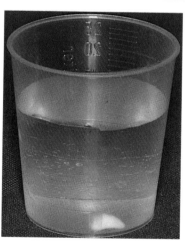

### Bonding of the fragment after 1 month
The temporary cover is removed and the fragment is fastened to a piece of sticky wax for ease of handling.

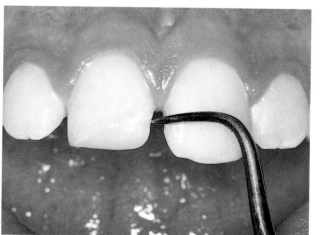 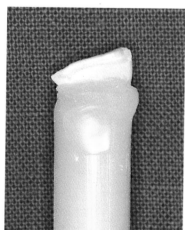

CROWN FRACTURES

### Preparing for bonding
Pulpal sensibility is monitored and the fracture surfaces (of the tooth and crown fragment) are cleansed with a pumice-water slurry and a rubber cup.

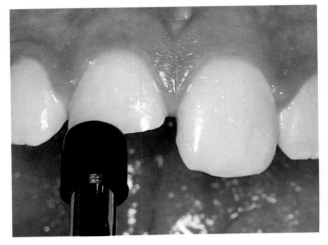 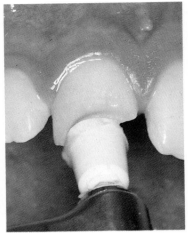

### Etching enamel
Enamel on both fracture surfaces as well as a 2-mm wide collar of enamel cervical and incisal to the fracture are etched for 30 seconds with 35% phosphoric acid gel, being sure that the etchant does not come in contact with dentin.

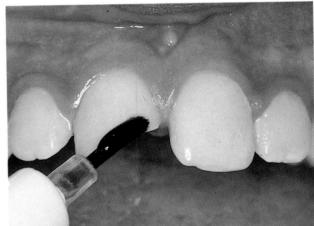 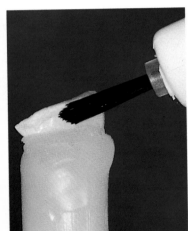

### Removal of the etchant
The fracture surfaces are rinsed thoroughly with a copious flow of water for 20 seconds.

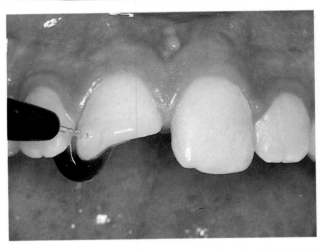 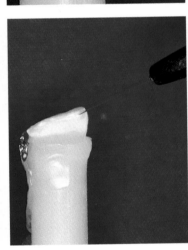

### Drying the fracture surfaces
The fracture surfaces are air-dried for 10 seconds. NOTE: To avoid entrapment of air in the dentinal tubules and a subsequent chalky mat discoloration of the fragment, the air stream must be directed parallel with the fracture surface and not perpendicular to it.

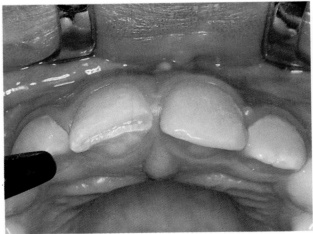 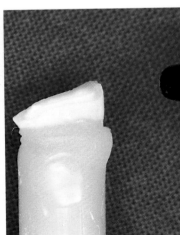

**Conditioning the dentin with EDTA and GLUMA®**

The fracture surfaces are conditioned with EDTA for 20 seconds; followed by 10 seconds water rinse and 10 seconds air drying. Thereafter 20 seconds GLUMA® and 10 seconds air drying.

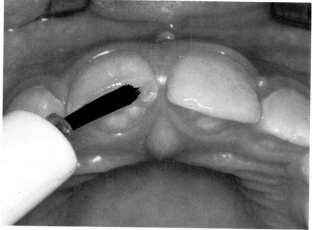 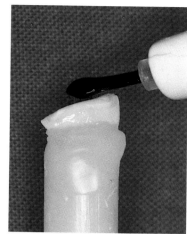

**Bonding the fragment**

The fracture surfaces are covered with a creamy mixture of a filled composite and its unfilled resin. After repositioning of the fragment, the composite is light-polymerized 60 seconds facially and 60 seconds orally.

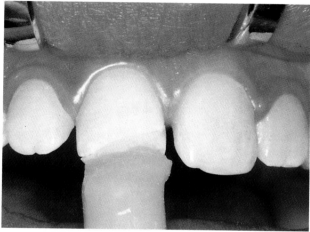 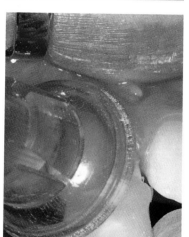

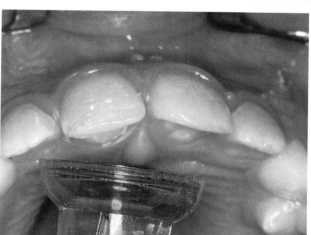 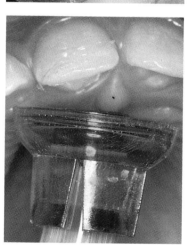

**Removal of surplus composite**

With a straight scalpel blade or composite finishing knives surplus composite is removed from the fracture site. The interproximal contacts are finished with finishing strips.

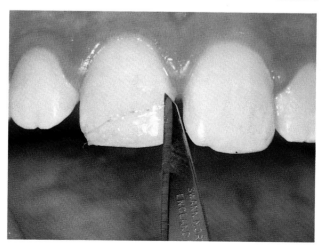 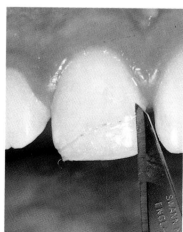

33

**Reinforcing the fracture site.**
A round diamond bur is used to create a "double chamfer" margin 1 mm coronally and apically to the fracture line. To achieve optimal esthetics, the chamfer follows an undulating path along the fracture line.

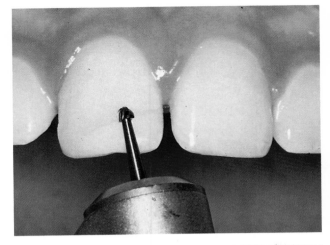
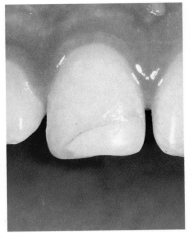

**Finishing the labial surface**
After restoring the labial aspect with composite, the restoration is contoured using abrasive discs.

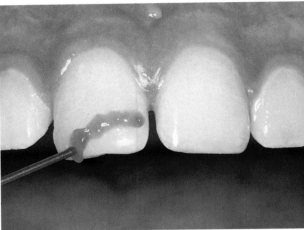
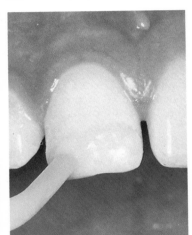

**Reinforcing the palatal aspect of the fracture**
The palatal aspect of the fracture is reinforced using the same procedure. Due to its position, esthetic consideration is less. The preparation can, therefore, follow the fracture line exactly.

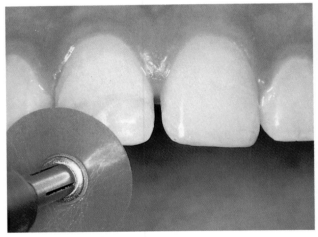
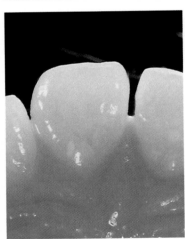

**The final restoration**
The condition 1 month after reattachment of the crown fragment.

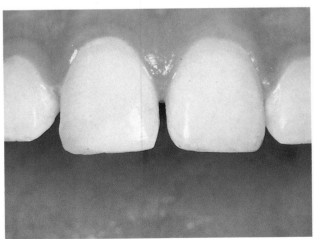
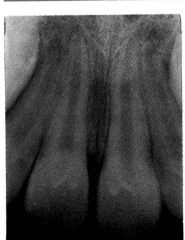

If necessary, the fragment is further hollowed out to accommodate the dressing over the hard tissue barrier and thus allow optimal repositioning of the fragment. Thereafter, bonding is performed as for uncomplicated fractures.

After bonding, patients are asked to use the teeth normally. Limitations in use, however, include all horizontal occlusal forces, e.g. pulling on chewy foods (hard breads, tough meats, toffees).

## Complicated crown fractures – pulpal considerations

Treatment of *pulp exposures* depends upon pulpal healing potential and the desirability of maintaining a vital pulp. Thus profound crown fracture of a mature tooth might dictate pulpal extirpation to permit restoration with a post-retained crown (Fig. 2.7).

In the event that a vital pulp is desired (as in young individuals) the following conditions must be fulfilled: 1.) The pulp should have been free of inflammation prior to injury; and 2.) any associated injury to the PDL must not have compromised the vascular supply to the pulp (Fig. 2.8).

If these conditions can be met, pulp capping and partial pulpotomy are the treatments of choice (Figs. 2.9 and 2.10). The choice between these two treatment procedures is unclear at present. Therefore, only a few *unsupported* guidelines can be given.

Fig. 2.7. Treatment of a complicated crown fracture by pulpal extirpation

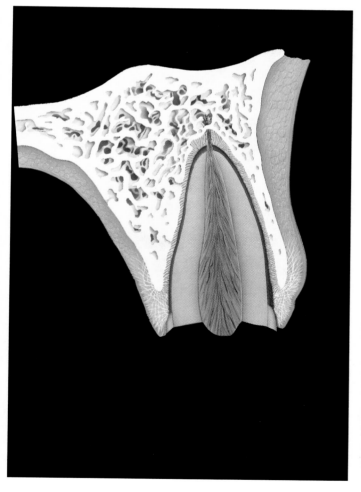
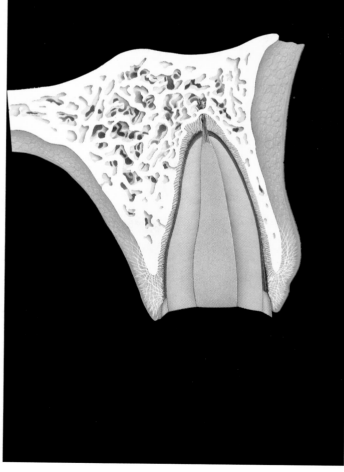

35

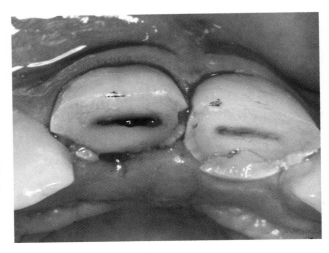

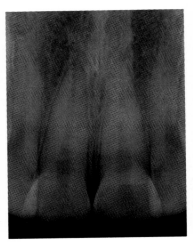

**Fig. 2.8. Evaluation of pulpal integrity following crown fracture**
The right central incisor was slightly loosened but not displaced at the time of injury (subluxation). The left central incisor was tender to percussion (concussion). The cyanotic, exposed pulp of the subluxated incisor reflects a compromised circulation following trauma. The exposed pulp of the left central incisor reflects intact circulation.

**Fig. 2.9. Treatment of a complicated crown fracture by pulp capping**

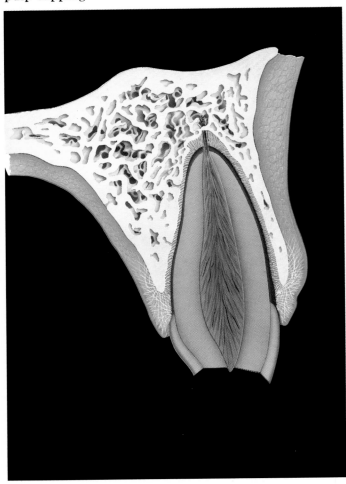

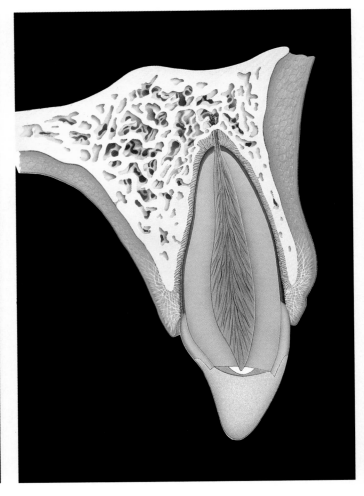

Thus, pulp capping should be used primarily for small exposures soon after injury (possibly within the first 24 hours) and where a restoration can be placed which provides a tight seal against bacterial invasion (Figs. 2.9 and 2.11).

In larger exposures with longer post-trauma intervals, a partial pulpotomy should be performed to a depth of 2 mm (Figs. 2.12 to 2.13). The amputation site should then be covered either with a hard setting calcium hydroxide cement, if later direct monitoring of the hard tissue barrier is not anticipated; or with pure calcium hydroxide, when later monitoring is desired. In the latter case, the perforation is covered with pure calcium hydroxide (e.g. Calasept®) and the exposed enamel and dentin is covered with a hard-setting calcium hydroxide cement (e.g. Dycal® or Life®). A temporary restoration is then placed which will ensure a tight seal against bacterial invasion of the healing pulp.

Fig. 2.10. Treatment of a complicated crown fracture by partial pulpotomy

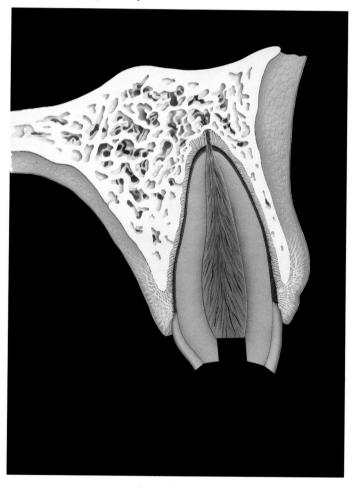
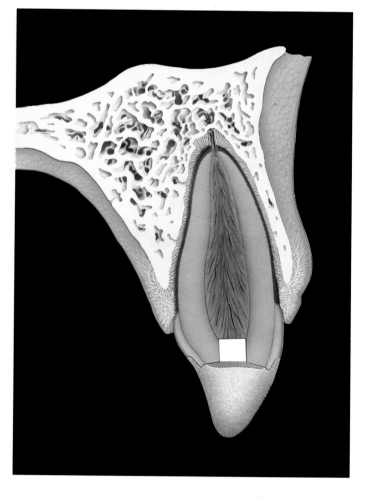

Three months after injury, the exposure site is uncovered. The amputation material as well as the necrotic pulp tissue immediately above the hard tissue barrier are removed. If the barrier appears intact, a bacteria-tight material is placed (e.g. glass ionomer cement or a dentin-bonded composite). The tooth can then be restored either with conventional composite buildup using the acid-etch technique or bonding of the original crown fragment using a dentin bonding system. The need for a hermetic seal seems relevant (although not proven), as all hard tissue barriers contain numerous vascular inclusions which allow direct bacterial invasion of the pulp.

Figs. 2.11-2.13 illustrate treatment of different types of crown fractures.

**Fig. 2.11. Treatment of a complicated crown fracture by pulp capping and a composite resin restoration**

This 12-year-old boy has suffered a crown fracture with a small pulp exposure. Note the good vascularity of the exposed pulp.

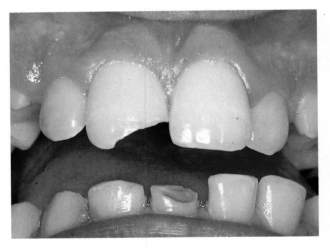
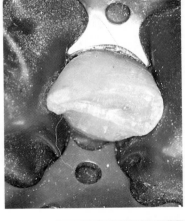

**Pulp capping**
After isolation with a rubber dam, the pulp exposure is covered with a calcium hydroxide paste (e.g. Calasept®). The remaining dentin is covered with a hard-setting calcium hydroxide cement, whereafter the tooth is restored with a composite. (Courtesy of Dr. M. Cvek, Eastman Dental Institute, Stockholm).

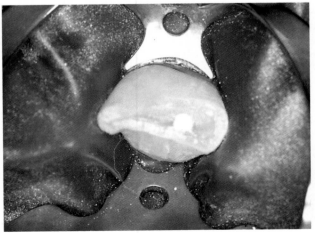
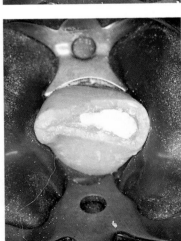

**Fig. 2.12. Treatment of a complicated crown fracture by pulpotomy and subsequent bonding of the crown fragment**

This 9-year-old boy has suffered a dental trauma 1 day previously. There is a small pulp exposure; pulpal vascularity appears intact.

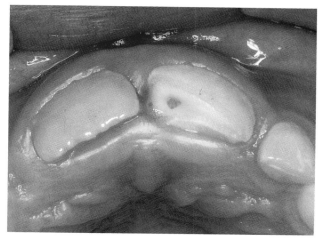 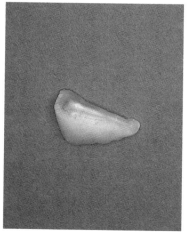

**Pulpotomy**

The tooth is isolated with a rubber dam and a pulpotomy is carried out using calcium hydroxide (i.e. Calasept®) and a glass ionomer cement as a cover.

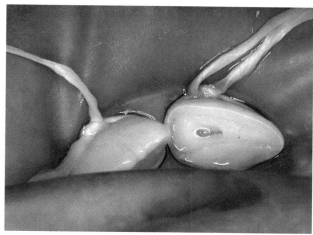 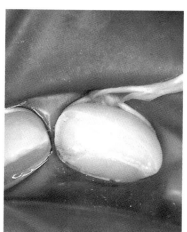

**Testing the fit of the fragment**

The fragment is tried in to ensure that the cover over the pulpotomy does not prevent correct repositioning of the fragment.

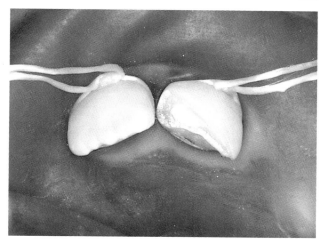 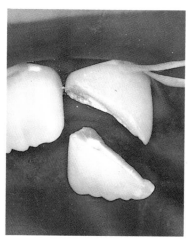

**Bonding the fragment**

The clinical and radiographic condition is shown 4 years after bonding. (Courtesy of Dr. M. Cvek, Eastman Dental Institute, Stockholm).

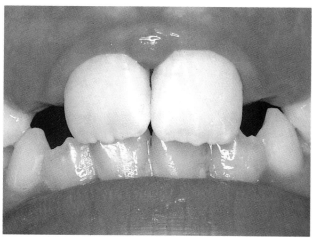 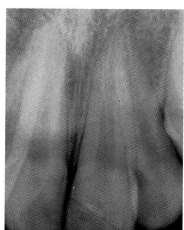

**Fig. 2.13. Complicated crown fracture treated by pulpotomy and composite restoration**
A 10-year-old boy who has suffered a crown fracture 2 days previously.

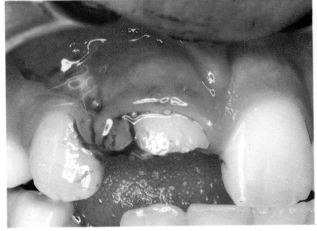 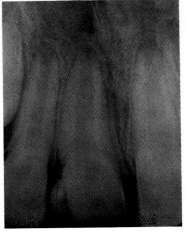

**Clinical condition**
A large pulp exposure is found.

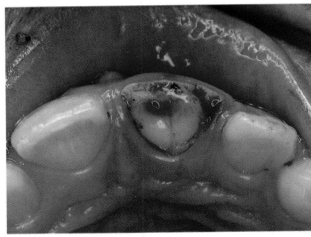 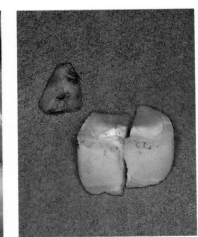

**Isolation with a rubber dam**
After administration of local anesthetic infiltration, the tooth is isolated with a rubber dam. An inverted diamond cone is used for the pulpotomy.

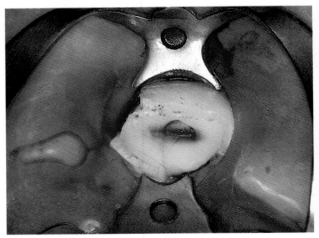 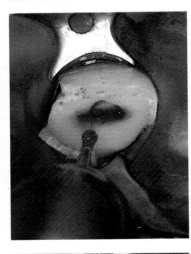

**Pulpotomy**
The pulpotomy is carried out to a depth of 2.0 mm, using a copious water spray from the airrotor, supplemented with an extra saline spray from a syringe.

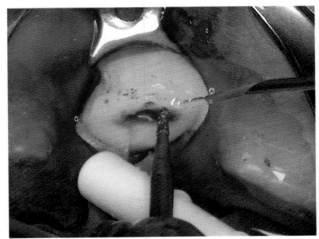 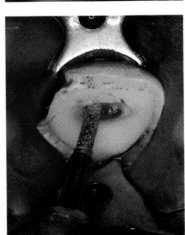

**Preparing the cavity**
The access cavity to the pulpotomy site should be boxlike, with a slight undercut in dentin.

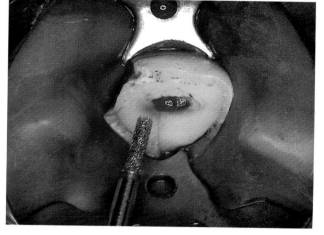
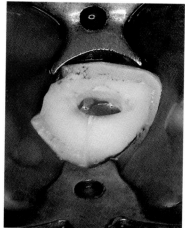

**Applying the amputation material**
Hemostasis is awaited. After some minutes, this will usually occur. Otherwise, slight pressure applied with a cotton pellet soaked in anesthetic solution with vasoconstrictor or calcium hydroxide can be used. After complete arrest of bleeding, calcium hydroxide paste (e.g. Calasept®) is placed on the pulpal wound.

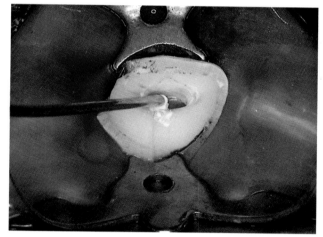
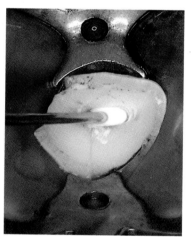

**Compressing the amputation material**
The material is compressed slightly using a cotton pellet. Thereafter, the entry site is covered with hard-setting calcium hydroxide cement.

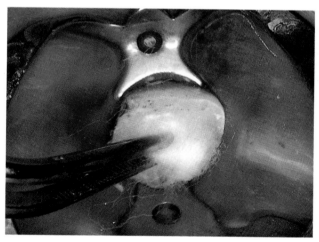
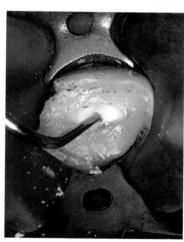

**Restoration**
The tooth in this case has been restored using a composite resin and a dentin bonding agent. (Courtesy of Dr. M. Cvek, Eastman Dental Institute, Stockholm).

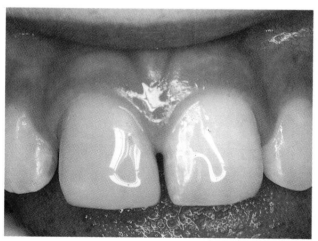
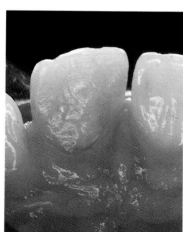

## Follow-up procedures

Crown fractured teeth should be followed in order to diagnose pulpal complications. A useful follow-up schedule is 1 and 2 months and 1 year after injury. Signs of pulp necrosis include loss of pulpal sensibility, coronal discoloration and periapical radiolucency. However, none of these signs is pathognomonic.

## General prognosis

The prognosis of crown fractures appears to depend primarily upon the presence of associated periodontal ligament injury and secondarily upon the extent of dentin exposed and the age of the pulp exposure (see Figs. 2.14 to 2.17).

Fig. 2.14. Pulpal healing after uncomplicated crown fracture in teeth with open apices according to type of luxation injury (after Andreasen & Andreasen 1989).

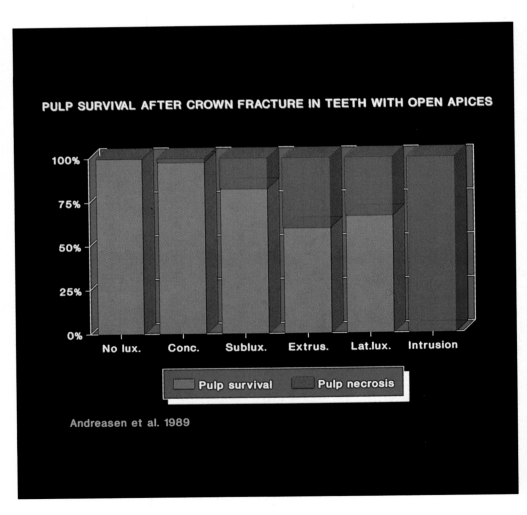

PULP SURVIVAL AFTER CROWN FRACTURE IN TEETH WITH OPEN APICES

Andreasen et al. 1989

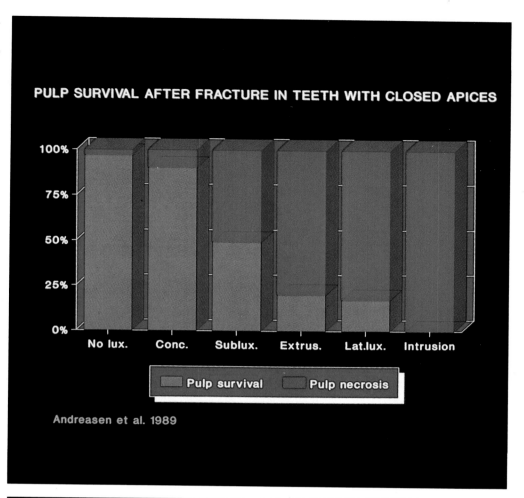

Fig. 2.16. **Pulpal healing after pulp capping** (after Ravn 1982).

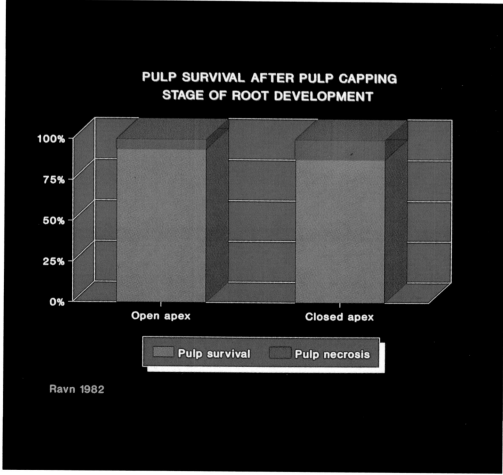

43

Fig. 2.17. **Pulpal healing after partial pulpotomy** (after Cvek 1978).

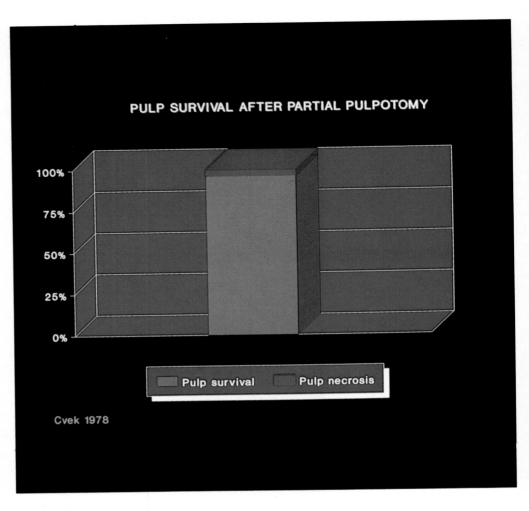

PULP SURVIVAL AFTER PARTIAL PULPOTOMY

Cvek 1978

## Essentials

Crown fractures represent a hazard to the pulp only if the following events have occurred:
– Associated periodontal ligament injury.
– Dentin or pulp exposure.

Treatment principles of crown fractures imply the following:
**Fractures of enamel**, depending on the site and extent of fracture:
– Selective grinding of the incisal edge and possibly of the adjacent tooth to reestablish symmetry.
– Acid-etch composite restoration.

### Fractures of enamel and dentin

A bacteria-tight cover of the exposed dentin should be established as soon after injury as possible. Dentinal coverage can include a calcium hydroxide base followed by dentin bonded composites and glass ionomer cements or bonding of the enamel-dentin crown fragment.

### Pulp exposures

The exposed pulp can usually be treated successfully (i.e. by the formation of a calcified bridge) under the following circumstances:

44

- No inflammation prior to trauma.
- Intact vascular supply after trauma.

Two treatment options exist:
- Pulp capping.
- Partial pulpotomy.

Which of these two treatment procedures is to be preferred has not yet been determined; however, the following conditions appear to favor *pulpotomy* rather than pulp capping:
- Long exposure period after trauma (i.e. more than 24 h).
- Large exposures (limit not established).
- Reduced vascularity due to a concomitant luxation injury.

Treatment procedures: *Pulp capping*
- Isolate the pulp exposure.
- Cover the pulp with a calcium hydroxide material (either hard-setting cement or pure calcium hydroxide paste).
- Restore the tooth either immediately with a bacteria-tight restoration; OR, after a 3-month period, where the exposure site is uncovered and the hard tissue barrier assessed. Thereafter, the hard tissue barrier is re-covered with a hard-setting calcium hydroxide cement, glass ionomer cement or a composite resin retained with a dentin bonding agent; and thereafter restored.

Treatment procedures: *Pulpotomy*
- Isolate the pulp exposure.
- Amputate the pulp to a level approximately 2 mm below the exposure site, or to where fresh bleeding is seen.
- If *immediate restoration* is desired, cover the exposure with a hard-setting calcium hydroxide cement (e.g. Dycal® or Life®).
- If *later assessment of the hard tissue barrier* is desired, cover the exposure with pure calcium hydroxide paste, cover the entire fracture surface (enamel and dentin) with a hard-setting calcium hydroxide cement and a temporary restoration for a period of 3 months. At that time, uncover the amputation site, remove the necrotic pulp tissue immediately above the hard tissue barrier and restore with a bacteria-tight restoration.

CROWN FRACTURES

# CHAPTER 3

# Crown-root fractures

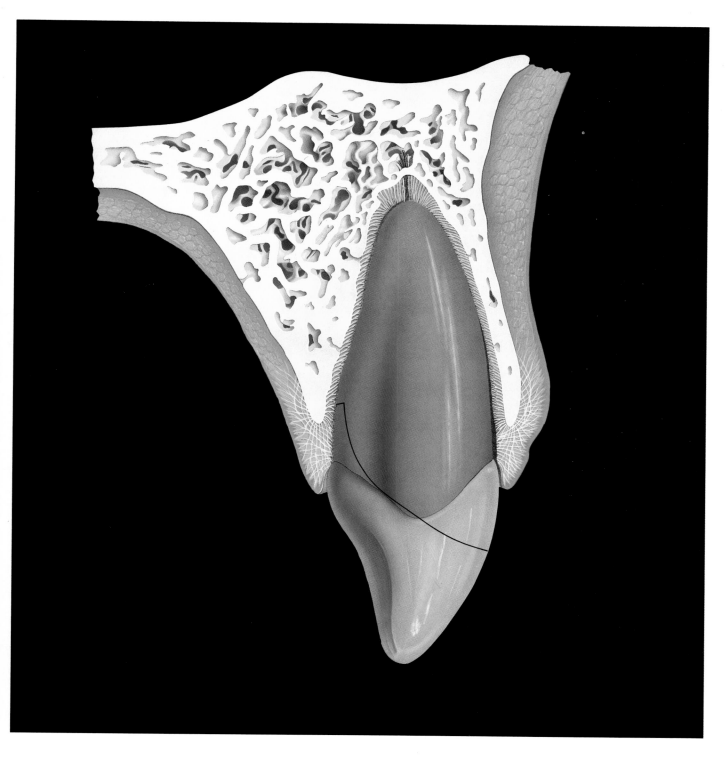

47

**Fig. 3.1. Fracture mechanism in a crown-root fracture**
The horizontal impact produces compression zones at the point of impact cervically on the palatal aspect and apically on the labial aspect of the root. The shearing stress zones which extend between the compression zones determine the course of the fracture.

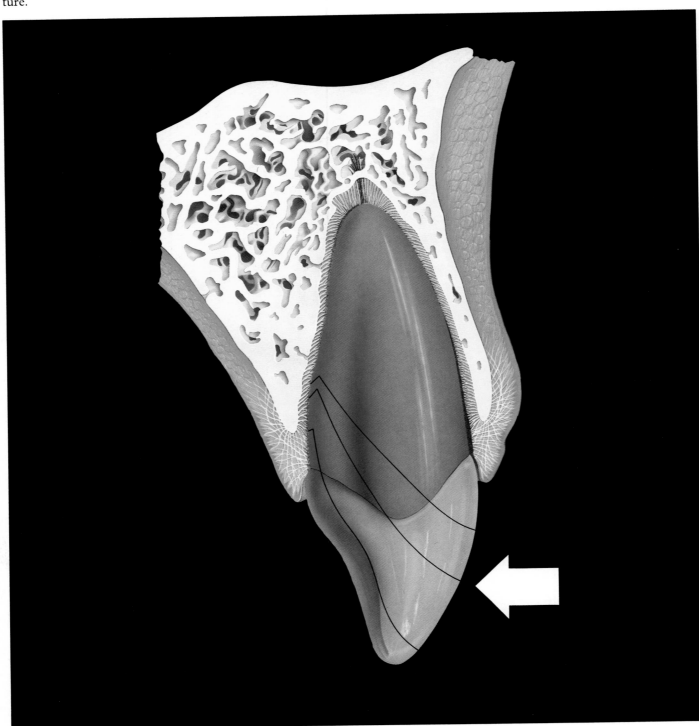

48

# Pattern of injury and diagnosis

This trauma entity is quite common and usually presents serious treatment problems due to the complex nature of the injury. Most of these fractures occur as the result of a horizontal impact. If the force of the impact exceeds the shearing strength of the hard dental tissues, a fracture will occur which initially follows the enamel rods of the labial surface of the crown and then takes an oblique course below the palatal gingival crest (Fig. 3.1). During its course through dentin, the fracture will often expose the pulp. The fracture line is usually single; but multiple fractures can occur, often commencing from the depth of the primary fracture.

A crown-root fracture left untreated usually results in pain from mastication due to movement of the coronal fragment; but is otherwise without symptoms.

The pathological events in case of no treatment comprise inflammatory changes in the pulp, periodontal ligament and the gingiva due to plaque accumulation in the line of fracture (Fig. 3.2).

The *clinical diagnosis* of a crown-root fracture is apparent when the coronal fragment is mobile (Fig. 3.2). The *radiographic diagnosis* is more difficult, at least with respect to its lingual extent, as the fracture line is usually perpendicular to the central radiographic beam (Fig. 3.2).

Fig. 3.2. **Clinical and radiographic diagnosis of a crown-root fracture**
The coronal fragment is mobile. The radiographs are not able to reveal the apical limit of the fracture.

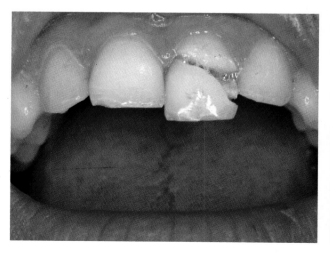 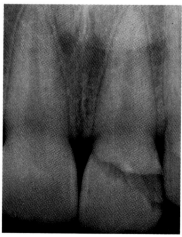

49

## Treatment

Most crown-root fractured teeth can be saved. In the following, various treatment procedures will be shown, including treatment indications, treatment principles and a cost-benefit analysis of their use.

## Removal of the coronal fragment with subsequent restoration above gingival level

**Treatment principle.** To allow the subgingival portion of the fracture to heal (presumably with formation of a long junctional epithelium), whereafter the coronal portion can be restored either by: bonding the original tooth fragment where the subgingival portion of the fragment has been removed using a dentin bonding system, a composite build-up using dentin and enamel bonding systems, or a crown restoration (Figs. 3.3 and 3.4).

**Indication.** This procedure should be limited to superficial fractures that do not involve the pulp.

**Treatment procedure.** The loose fragment is removed as soon as possible after injury. Rough edges along the fracture surface below the gingiva may be smoothed with a chisel. The remaining

Fig. 3.3. Removal of the coronal fragment and supragingival restoration

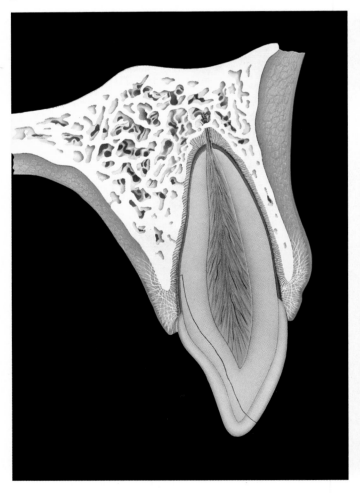 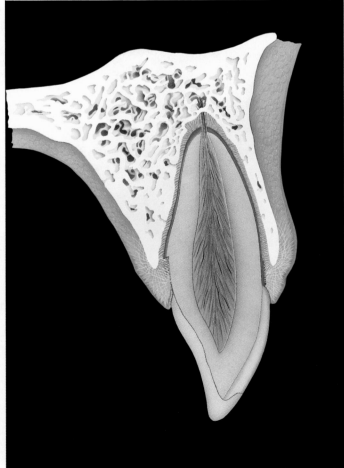

50

crown is covered with a temporary crown whose margin ends supragingivally. Once gingival healing is seen (after 2-3 weeks), the crown can be restored.

**Cost-benefit.** The method is easily followed and treatment time is short. However, the long-term effect with respect to the pulp and periodontium remains to be documented.

**Fig. 3.4. Removal of the coronal fragment and supragingival restoration**
This 16-year-old girl has suffered a crown-root fracture which has exposed the palatal root surface. The clinical condition is shown after gingivectomy.

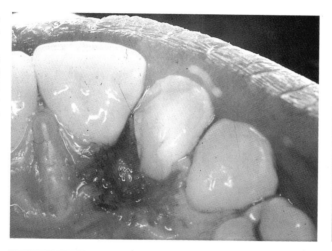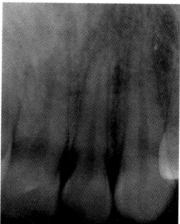

**Condition 1 week after gingivectomy**
The palatal fragment has been removed and the exposed root dentin smoothed with a bur; the exposed dentin covered with calcium hydroxide and a temporary crown. Two weeks later creeping reattachment is seen and the palatal of the crown restored with a dentin bonded composite resin restoration.

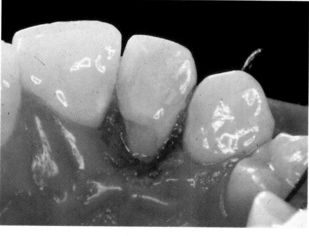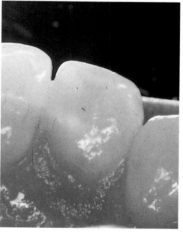

**Follow-up**
Clinical and radiographic condition 4 years after treatment. (Courtesy of Dr. B. Malmgren, Eastman Institute, Stockholm, Sweden)

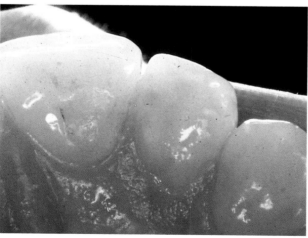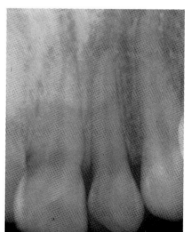

CROWN-ROOT FRACTURES

## Removal of the coronal fragment supplemented by gingivectomy and osteotomy and subsequent restoration with a post-retained crown

**Treatment principle.** To convert the subgingival fracture to a supragingival fracture with the help of gingivectomy and osteotomy (Fig. 3.5).

**Indication.** Should only be used where the surgical technique does not compromise the esthetic result, i.e. only the palatal aspect of the fracture must be exposed in this manner.

**Treatment procedure.** The coronal fragment is removed and a gingivectomy and osteotomy are performed. Bone is removed 2 mm below the level of the fracture (Fig. 3.5). At the same time, the pulp is extirpated. The root filling can be placed at the same session or at a later appointment. Once the root filling is complete, an impression is taken for a post-retained crown.

**Cost-benefit.** Treatment time is short. However, long-term follow-up of these restorations has shown a slight tendency for the crowns to migrate labially. Furthermore, the palatal gingiva was often hyperplastic and inflamed despite good adaptation of the crown margins.

52

**Fig. 3.5. Removal of the coronal fragment and surgical exposure of the fracture**
Clinical and radiographic appearance of a complicated crown-root fracture.

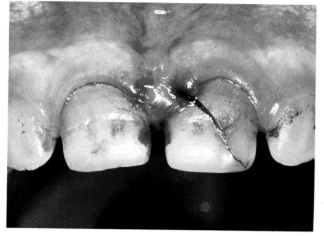 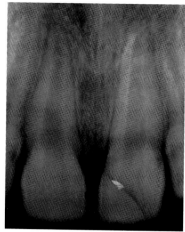

**Exposing the fracture site**
The coronal fragment is removed. A combined gingivectomy and osteotomy expose the fracture surface.

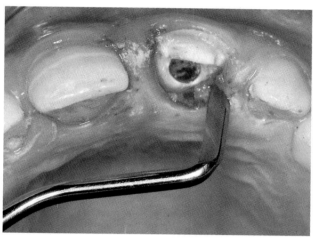 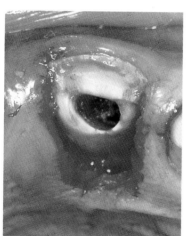

**Constructing a post-retained crown**
After taking an impression, a post-retained full crown is fabricated.

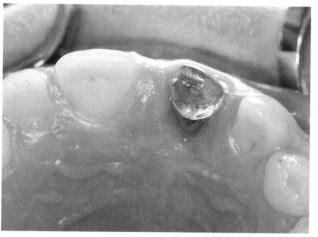 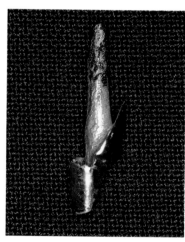

**The finished restoration**
The clinical and radiographic condition 2 months after insertion of the crown.

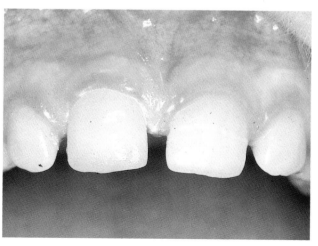 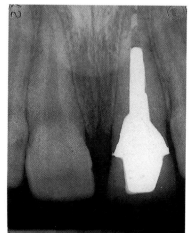

CROWN-ROOT FRACTURES

## Removal of the coronal fragment and surgical extrusion of the root

**Treatment principle.** To surgically move the fracture to a supragingival position (Fig. 3.6).

**Indication.** Should only be used where the root portion is long enough to accommodate a post-retained crown.

**Treatment.** As soon after injury as possible, the coronal fragment is removed (Fig. 3.7). The apical fragment is luxated with an elevator and removed with forceps. The pulp can be extirpated at this time. The root is then moved into a more coronal position and secured in that position with sutures and/or a splint. In case of palatally inclined fractures, 180° rotation can often imply that only slight extrusion is necessary to accommodate crown preparation. After 2-3 weeks, the tooth can be treated endodontically. After another 1-2 months, the tooth can be restored with a post-retained crown.

**Cost-benefit.** Several clinical studies have indicated that this is a safe and rapid method for the treatment of crown-root fractures. However, pulp vitality must be sacrificed.

Fig. 3.6. Removal of the coronal fragment and surgical extrusion of the root

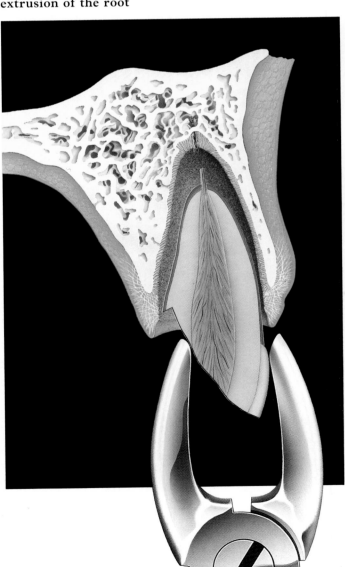
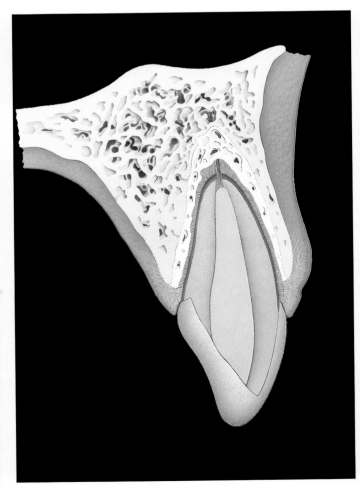

**Fig. 3.7. Removal of the coronal fragment and surgical extrusion of the root**
A complicated crown-root fracture in a 13-year-old boy.
The loose fragment is stabilized immediately after injury with a temporary crown and bridge material using the acid-etch technique.

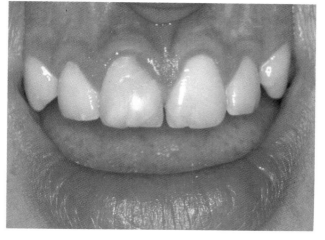
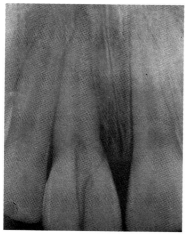

**Incision of the PDL**
Using a specially contoured surgical blade, the PDL is incised as far apically as possible.

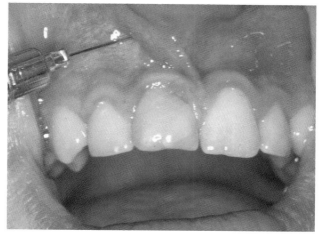
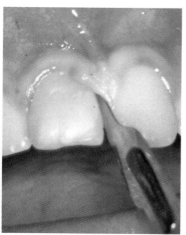

**Luxation of the root**
The root is then luxated with a narrow elevator which is placed at the mesiopalatal and distopalatal corners respectively.

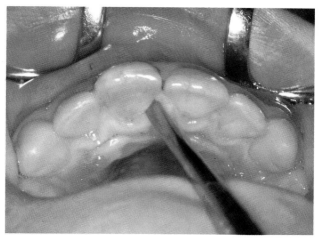
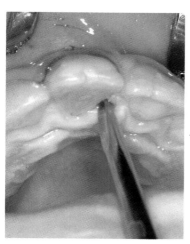

**Extracting the root**
The root is extracted and inspected for additional fractures.

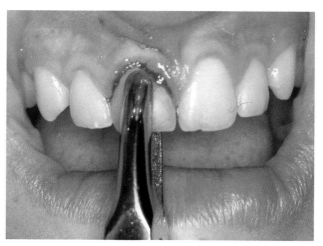
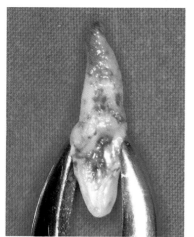

### Replanting the apical fragment

The root is tried in different positions in order to establish where the fracture is optimally exposed yet with minimal extrusion. In this instance, optimal repositioning was achieved by rotating the root 45°.

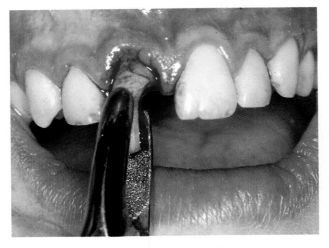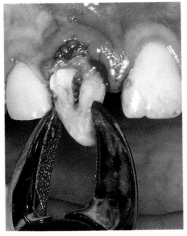

### Stabilization of the apical fragment during healing

The root is splinted to adjacent teeth. The pulp is extirpated and the access cavity to the root canal closed.

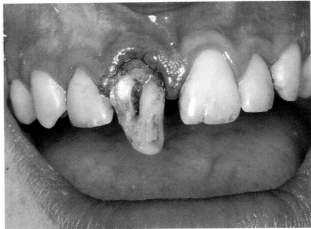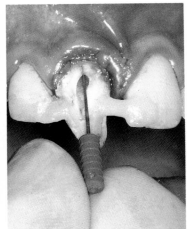

### Root filling

Two weeks after initial treatment, endodontic therapy can be continued, in the form of an interim dressing with calcium hydroxide. The root canal is obturated with gutta percha and sealer as far apically as possible 1 month after surgical extrusion.

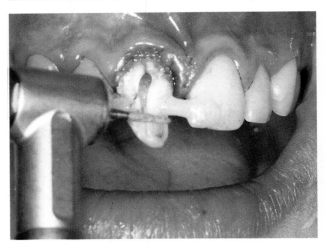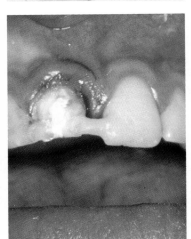

### Completion of the restoration

Two months after surgical extrusion, healing has occurred and it is possible to complete the restoration.

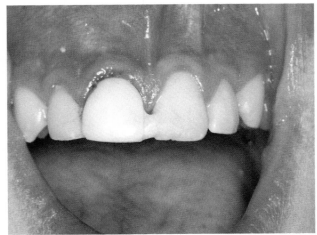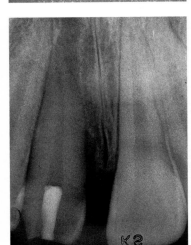

## Removal of the coronal fragment and subsequent orthodontic extrusion of the root

**Treatment principle.** To orthodontically move the fracture to a supragingival position (Fig. 3.8).

**Indication.** The same as for surgical extrusion, but is more time-consuming.

**Treatment.** The coronal fragment is removed, the pulp extirpated and the root canal filled (Fig. 3.9). Alternatively, the endodontic therapy can be performed prior to the removal of the coronal fragment (i.e. while the coronal fragment is temporarily splinted to the adjacent teeth). This might facilitate the endodontic procedure. Alternatively, a pulp capping or pulpotomy may be performed, a situation which is indicated if root formation is not complete (Fig. 3.10). Thereafter, orthodontic traction is applied to either a bracket fastened to the labial surface of the fragment or to a hook cemented into the root canal. The root is then extruded over a period of 2-3 weeks. The gingiva will follow

Fig. 3.8. Removal of the coronal fragment and orthodontic extrusion of the root

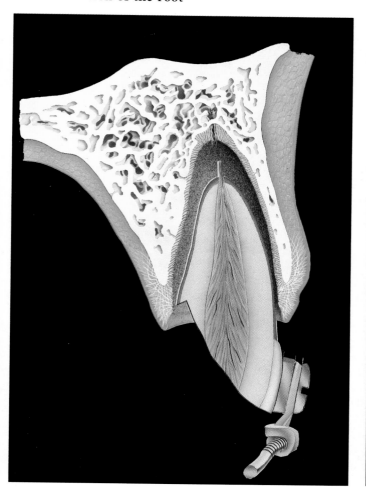 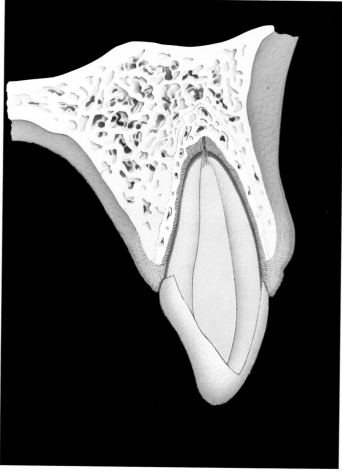

57

the path of the extruding root, thus necessitating a gingivectomy once extrusion is complete. The tooth is then retained for 2-3 months, whereafter it can be restored with a composite build-up or a post-retained crown.

**Cost-benefit.** The procedure is slow and cumbersome. However, it provides excellent esthetic results and the gingival health appears to be optimal. Pulp vitality can be saved if indicated.

## Follow-up procedures

Each procedure bears with it routine monitoring of periodontal status clinically and radiographically. Follow-up intervals should be at 2 months after completed treatment and 1 year after injury.

## General prognosis

See the individual treatment procedures.

Fig. 3.9. Removal of the coronal fragment, pulp extirpation and orthodontic extrusion
A complicated crown root fracture in a 13-year-old boy.

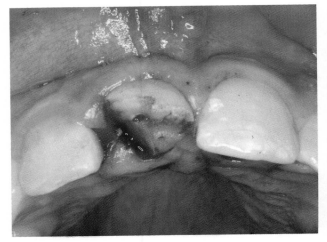 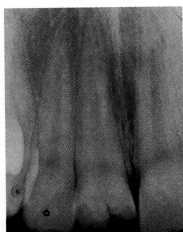

**Endodontic treatment**
The pulp has been extirpated. After a period with a calcium hydroxide interim dressing, the canal is filled with gutta percha and a sealer.

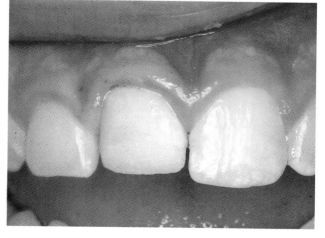
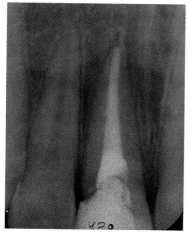

**Applying extrusion appliances**
Two premolars and the canine are used as anchorage for the orthodontic appliances.

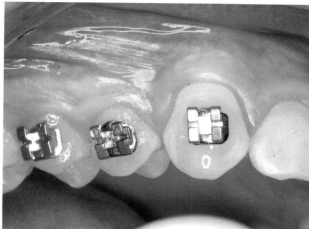
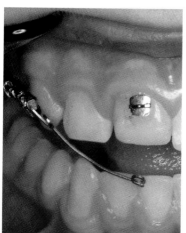

**Orthodontic extrusion**
The tooth is extruded quickly over a period of 2-3 weeks in order to prevent coronal migration of marginal bone.

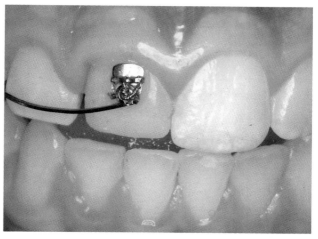
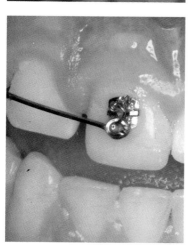

**Condition 1 year after extrusion**
The root has been extruded and the dentin covered with glass ionomer cement and then restored with composite (Courtesy of Dr. B. Malmgren and E. Köndell, Eastman Dental Institute, Stockholm).

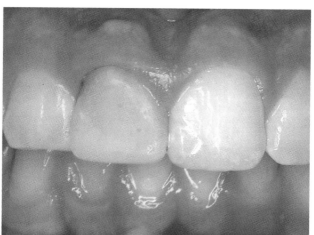
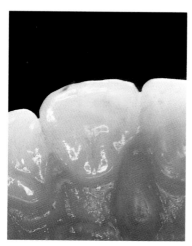

### Fig. 3.10. Removal of the coronal fragment, pulpotomy and orthodontic extrusion

A complicated crown-root fracture of a mandibular central incisor in a 14-year-old girl.

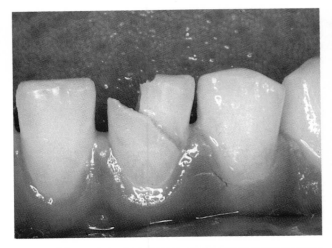

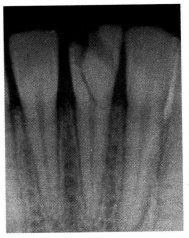

### Removing the loose fragment

The coronal fragment is removed, revealing a large pulp exposure. However, pulpal vascularity appears intact.

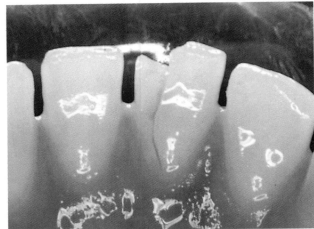

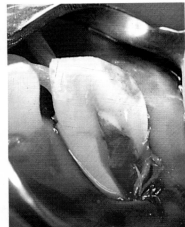

### Pulpotomy

A pulpotomy is performed. The level of amputation is placed at the cervical area, and the tooth temporarily restored with glass ionomer cement.

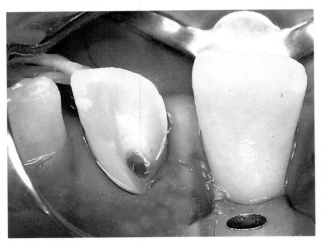

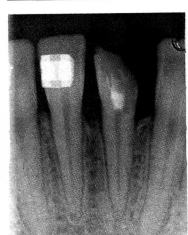

### Orthodontic extrusion

After verification of a hard tissue closure at the amputation site, the tooth is extruded using an orthodontic appliance.

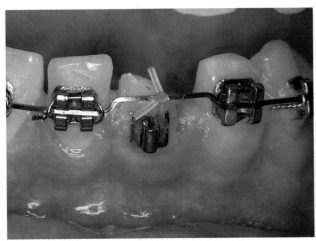

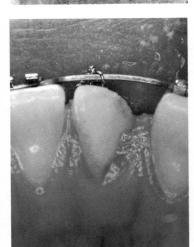

60

**Extrusion complete**
After extrusion and a fibrotomy the tooth is retained using an acid-etch retainer employing glass fiber and composite resin.

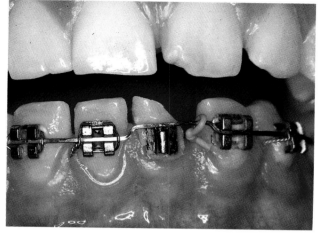

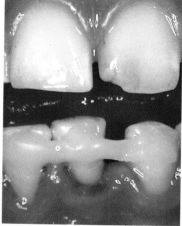

**Restoration completed**
The tooth has been restored using a combination of glass ionomer cement and composite resin (Courtesy of Dr. B. Malmgren & K. Ridell, Eastman Dental Institute, Stockholm).

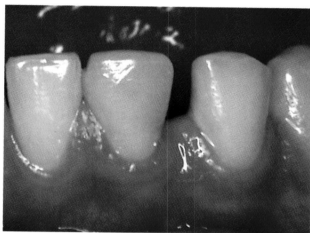

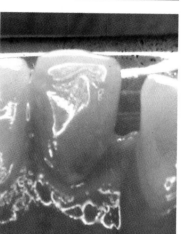

## Essentials

Crown-root fractures may or may not involve the pulp.

Clinical diagnosis depends upon mobility of the coronal fragment. Radiographic diagnosis, however, is uncertain as it is usually impossible to determine the oral extent of fracture.

Treatment principles include the following
- **Removal of the coronal fragment and supragingival restoration** (e.g. by bonding the original crown fragment after removing the subgingival portion, with composite build-up or a crown) in order to permit subgingival healing, presumably with a long junctional epithelium.
- **Removal of the coronal fragment supplemented by gingivectomy and/or osteotomy,** in order to convert the subgingival fracture surface to supragingival in situations where esthetics permit; thereafter, restoration (e.g. with a post-retained crown).
- **Removal of the coronal fragment and surgical or orthodontic extrusion of the root,** to move the fracture surface to a more optimal location for final restoration.

61

# Root fracture

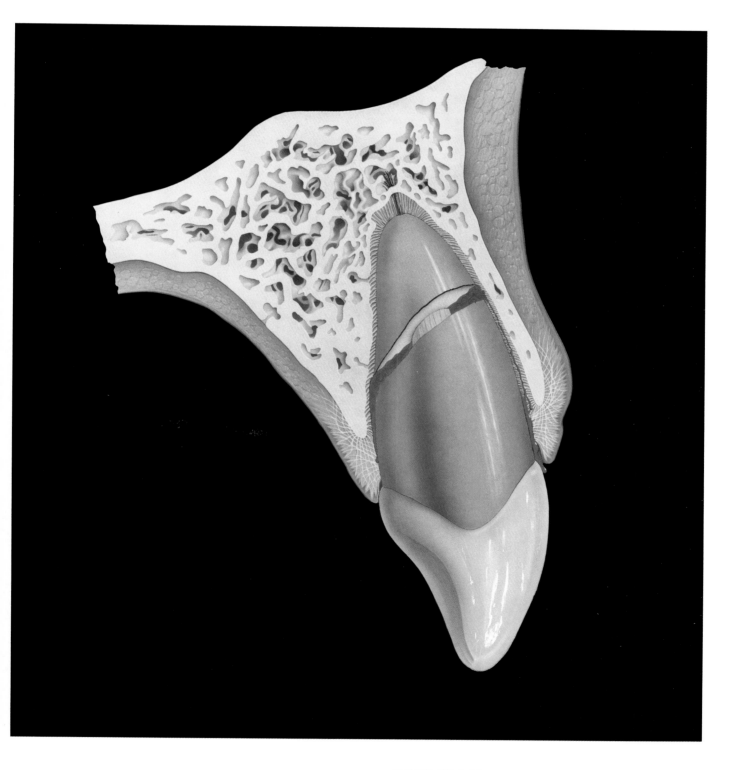

ROOT FRACTURE

**Fig. 4.1. Mechanism of root fracture**
A frontal impact displaces the tooth lingually and results in a root fracture and displacement of the coronal fragment. This results in both pulp and PDL damage.

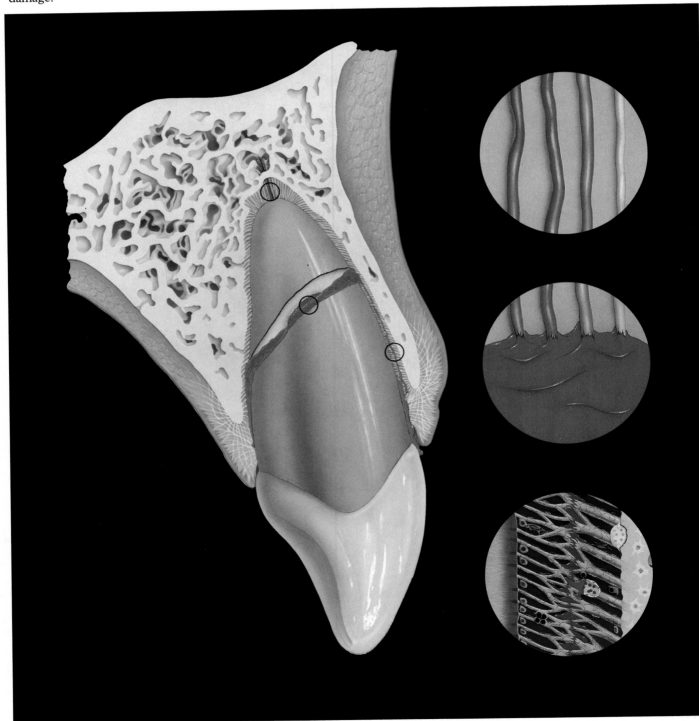

64

# Pattern of injury and diagnosis

Root fractures are relatively uncommon injuries, but represent complex healing patterns due to concomitant injury to the pulp, periodontal ligament, dentin and cementum. The fracture usually results from a horizontal impact. Fractures in the apical- and middle-thirds of the root normally take an oblique course, being placed more apically on the labial aspect than on the palatal (Fig. 4.1). A rather steep radiographic exposure is needed for optimal fracture detection in these locations. However, as the level of fracture approaches the cervical one-third, the direction of fracture changes, being more or less perpendicular to the fractures in the apical- and middle-thirds. These fractures obviously require a different angulation of the central beam in order to be detected radiographically. Thus, more than one radiographic exposure is necessary to ensure detection of all root fractures.

The frontal impact tends to force the coronal fragment palatally and in a slightly extruded direction. In this way the pulp may be stretched, but may or may not be severed, due to its inherent elasticity.

The healing events which subsequently take place are primarily dependent upon two conditions: whether the pulp is severed and whether bacteria have invaded the fracture line. If the pulp is intact after injury, a dentin callus is formed between the two fragments after some weeks, whereafter the peripheral aspect of

**Fig. 4.2. Hard tissue healing after pulpal injury**
The pulp is ruptured at the level of the fracture. Fracture healing with ingrowth of cells originating from the apical half of the pulp ensures hard tissue healing of the fracture.

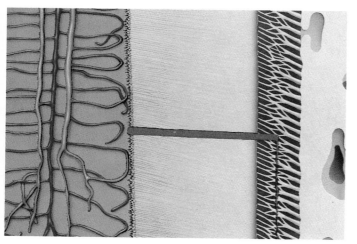
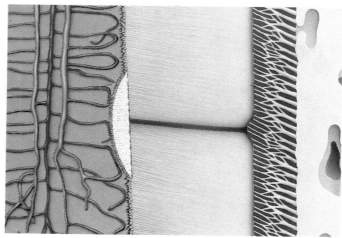

**Fig. 4.3. Connective tissue healing after pulpal injury**
The pulp is ruptured at the level of the fracture. Healing is dominated by ingrowth of cells originating from the periodontal ligament and results in interposition of connective tissue between the two fragments.

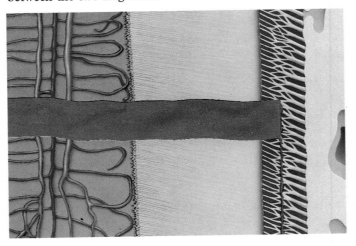 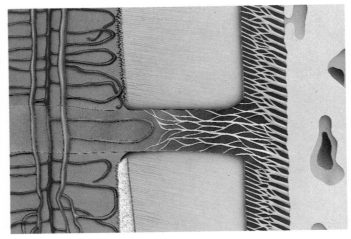

**Fig. 4.4. Non-healing due to infection in the line of fracture**
Infection occurs in the avascular coronal aspect of the pulp. Granulation tissue is soon formed which originates from the apical pulp and periodontal ligament. Accumulation of tissue between the two fragments causes separation of the fragments and loosening of the coronal fragment.

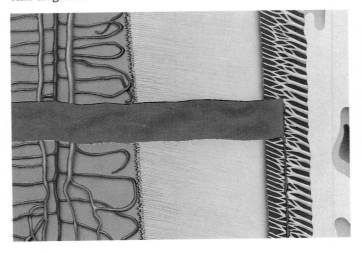 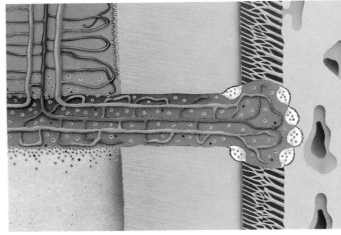

the fracture is healed by cementum deposition, a process which can take place over a period of several years (Fig. 4.2).

If the pulp has been ruptured, revascularization of the coronal aspect of the pulp has to take place prior to fracture healing. The exact nature of this process is not yet known. But it is suspected that two events can take place; namely, invasion of cells derived from the apical pulp or invasion of cells from the periodontal ligament (Fig. 4.3). Depending upon the source of cells entering the coronal pulp canal, healing of the fracture will take place by either union with hard tissue or by interposition of connective tissue (from the periodontal ligament) respectively.

In the event that bacteria gain access to the coronal pulp in its avascular condition, healing of the pulp is impossible and an accumulation of granulation tissue between root fragments will result as a response to the infected coronal aspect of the pulp (Fig. 4.4).

## Treatment

To facilitate pulpal and periodontal ligament healing, it is considered essential (although not proven) that a displaced coronal fragment be optimally repositioned. Furthermore, that splinting be maintained for a 3-month period in order to permit maximum stability of the hard tissue callus (Fig. 4.5). In Figs. 4.6 and 4.7, repositioning and splinting of root fractures with different types of displacement (luxation) of the coronal fragment are demonstrated.

## Follow-up procedures

Sensibility testing and radiographic examination should be performed 3 weeks, 6 weeks and 3 months after injury (see Appendix 4, page 161).

**Radiographic guidelines.** Recent clinical studies have indicated that certain radiographic findings can be used as predictors for root fracture healing.

**Resorption within the root canal** originating at the fracture line is apparently a stage in healing following pulpal damage after trauma. This has been found to be followed by later mineralization events and healing by interposition of connective tissue. This condition does not require treatment, but does require regular follow-up control.

**Resorption within bone** at the level of the fracture line is, however, an indicator of pulp necrosis, usually of the coronal fragment. This condition requires endodontic therapy; that is, extirpation of the the necrotic coronal pulp, interim dressing with a calcium hydroxide paste and finally gutta percha root filling.

**Pulp canal obliteration** of the coronal and apical root canals indicates a response to pulpal injury and subsequent healing by interposition of connective tissue between fragments.

Fig. 4.5. **Principles for treatment of root fractures**
Treatment of root fractures consists of complete repositioning and firm, immobile splinting, preferably with a passively applied splint (see text), until a hard tissue callus is formed.

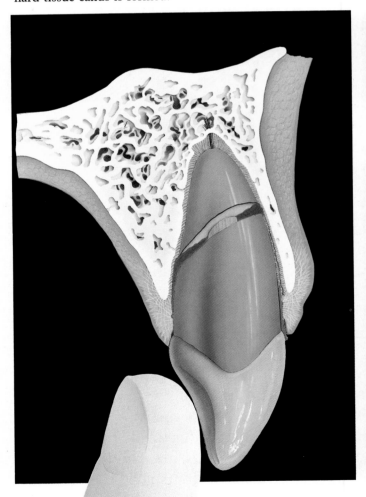
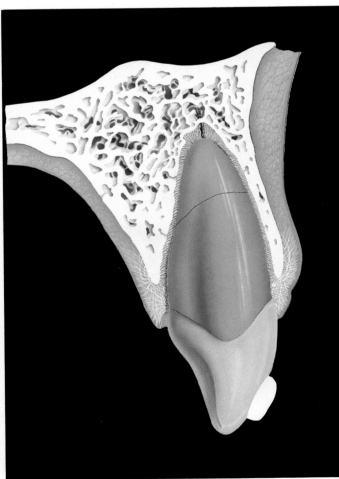

CHAPTER 4

## Fig. 4.6. Treatment of a laterally luxated root fracture

This 13-year-old boy received a horizontal blow to the right maxillary central incisor.

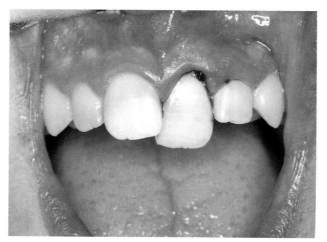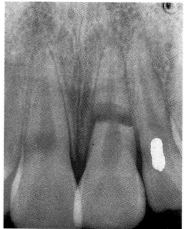

### Examining the tooth

The tooth reacts to SENSIBILITY TESTING, indicating an intact vascular supply. There is a high metallic sound elicited by the PERCUSSION TEST, indicating lateral luxation of the coronal fragment. The tooth is locked firmly in its displaced position, confirming the luxation diagnosis.

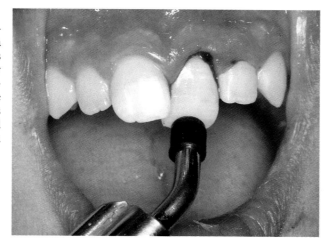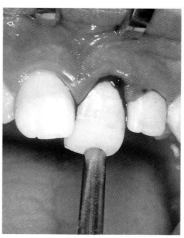

### Repositioning

Because of the force necessary to reposition a laterally luxated tooth, local anesthesia is administered prior to repositioning. Firm pressure is applied to the facial bone plate at the fracture level in order to displace the coronal fragment out of its alveolar "lock." This is followed by horizontal (forward) pressure at the palatal aspect of the incisal edge, which repositions the coronal fragment into its original position.

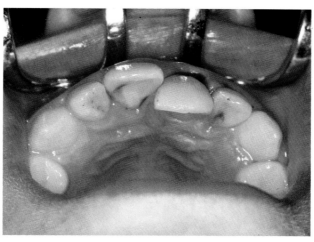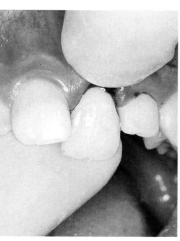

### Verifying repositioning

The correct position of the coronal fragment is confirmed radiographically.

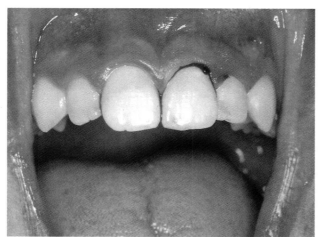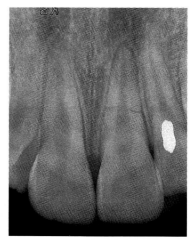

69

ROOT FRACTURE

**Fixation procedure**

The acid-etch technique and a temporary crown and bridge material is used. Phosphoric acid gel is applied for 30 seconds to the facial surfaces of the injured and adjacent non-injured teeth. The tooth surfaces are then rinsed thoroughly with a stream of water for 20-30 seconds and blown dry. A mat enamel surface indicates adequate etching.

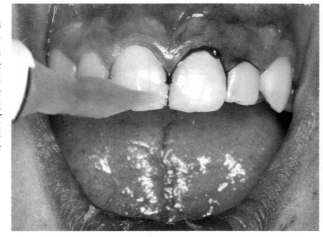
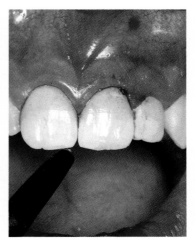

**Applying the splinting material**

A composite or unfilled resin is applied to the etched enamel surfaces. The bulk of the material should be placed on the mesial and distal corners of the traumatized and the adjacent, non-injured incisors. After setting, any irregularity in the surface is removed with abrasive discs or a scalpel blade proximally.

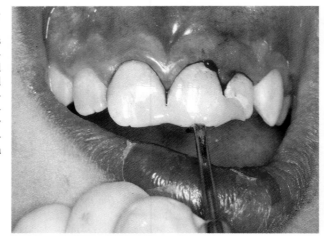
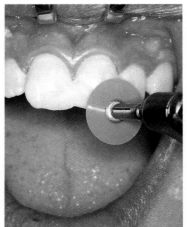

**Removing the splint**

The healing events are monitored radiographically 1-, 2- and 3 months after injury. If, after these periods, the tooth reacts to sensibility testing and there is no sign of infection in the bone at the level of the fracture, the splint may be removed.

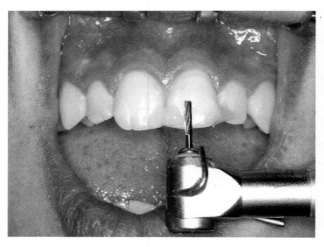
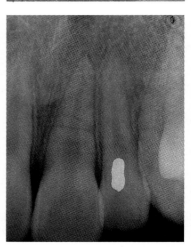

**One year after injury**

The tooth reacts normally to sensibility testing and the radiograph shows increasing radioopacity of the fracture line.

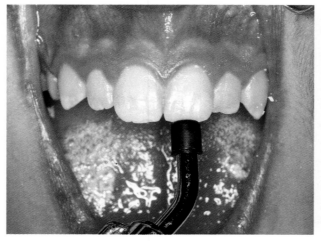
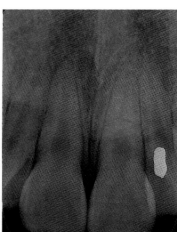

70

### Fig. 4.7. Treatment of a severely extruded root fracture

This 20-year-old woman has suffered a frontal blow to the central incisor, resulting in extreme displacement of the coronal fragment.

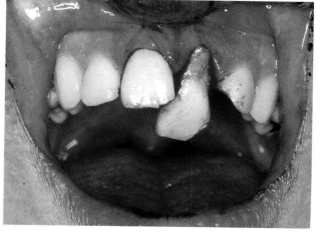 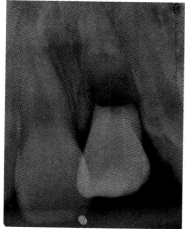

### Examining the displaced coronal fragment

After cleansing of the exposed root surface with saline, it can be seen that the coronal fragment has been forced past the cervical margin of the labial bone plate. The stretched pulp is seen within the socket area.

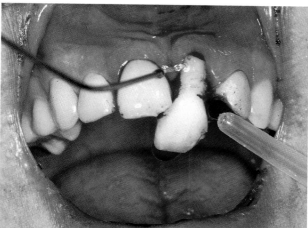 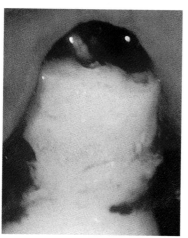

### Repositioning

After local anesthetic infiltration, the coronal fragment is repositioned. To guide the root fragment into place, an amalgam carver is inserted beneath the cervical bone margin and used like a shoe horn.

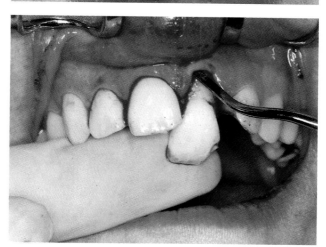 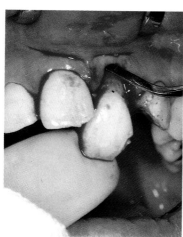

### Splinting

The acid-etch technique is employed once optimal repositioning has been verified radiographically. The labial surfaces are etched and a splinting material (composite or unfilled resin) is applied. The patient is given penicillin (2 million IU daily for 4 days) to safeguard healing.

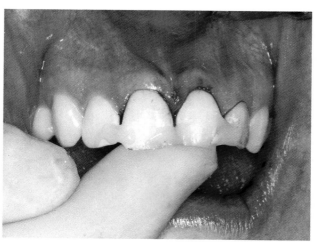 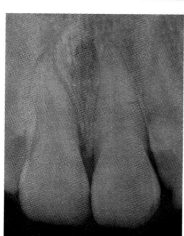

### Diagnosing healing complications

Negative pulpal sensibility, increased separation between fragments as seen radiographically after 3-4 weeks, together with periradicular radiolucencies (arrows) indicate pulp necrosis in the coronal fragment.

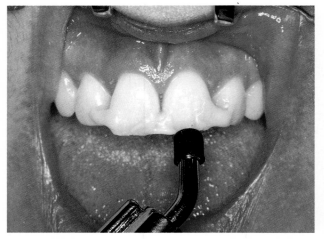
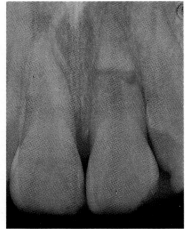

### Endodontic treatment of the coronal fragment

A rubber dam is placed over the splinted teeth by punching three adjacent holes and connecting them with a scissors' cut. In that way, the splinted teeth can be isolated. The rubber dam can be held in place by wedging a small piece of rubber dam material between the last tooth in the splint and the next unsplinted tooth.

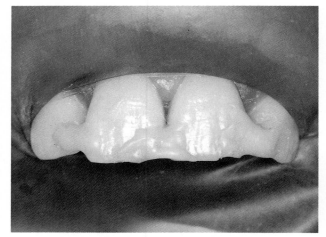
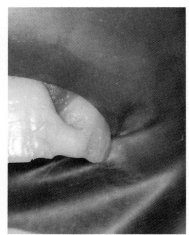

### Entering the pulp chamber

After disinfecting the palatal surface of the tooth with a bactericidal solution (e.g. a combination of hydrogen peroxide and chlorhexidine-cetrimonium), an access cavity is prepared and the pulp extirpated.

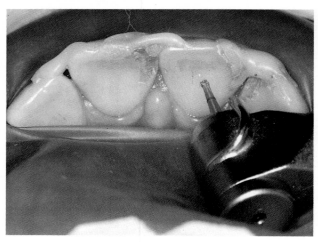
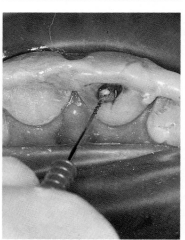

### Extirpation of the coronal pulp

A barbed broach is inserted into the coronal aspect of the root canal, short of the fracture line, and the pulp extirpated.

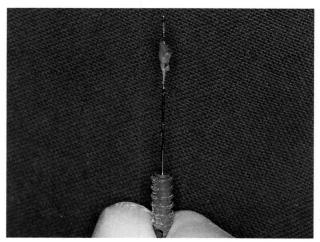
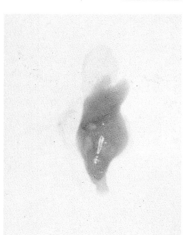

**Preparation of the root canal**
The root canal is rinsed with 2% sodium hypochlorite. A relatively large file is inserted in the root canal as a guide to the level of amputation. A slight pain response will be elicited from the patient when vital tissue at the fracture level is reached. This level should NEVER be exceeded during mechanical preparation.

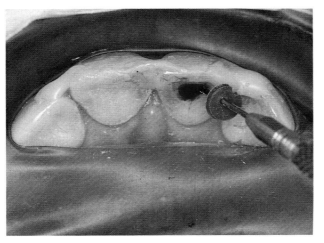 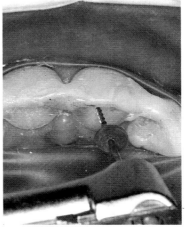

**Obturating the root canal**
To induce hard tissue closure of the coronal aspect of the "fracture foramen," calcium hydroxide paste (e.g. Calasept®, Scandia Dental) is used initially as a root canal dressing. The paste is carried into the root canal with a lentulo spiral and condensed with paper points.

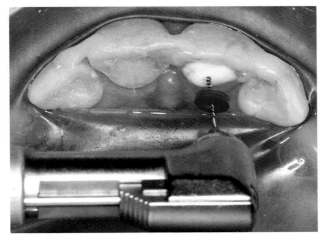 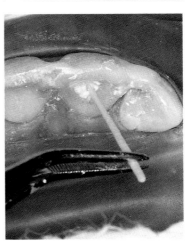

**Sealing the root canal**
A small cotton pellet is placed in the coronal aspect of the canal, approximately 2 mm from the oral surface of the access cavity. The margins of the access cavity are cleansed of calcium hydroxide paste. Thereafter, the cavity is sealed with fortified zinc oxide eugenol cement or glass ionomer cement. A radiograph is taken upon completion of treatment. It should be noted that calcium hydroxide paste has the same radioopacity as dentin.

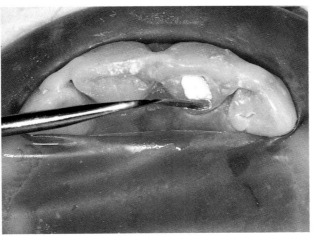 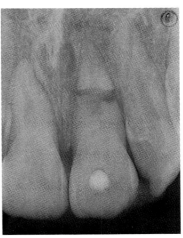

**Follow-up**
The calcium hydroxide treatment is repeated 1 month after initial treatment. Thereafter, radiographic controls were performed after 6 months and 1 year. At this time, a hard tissue barrier was formed and endodontic treatment then completed by insertion of a gutta percha root filling. The clinical and radiographic situation is shown 1 year after injury where the tooth has been restored with a composite resin build-up and the root canal filled with gutta percha.

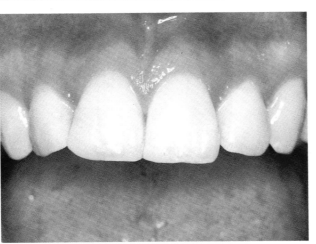 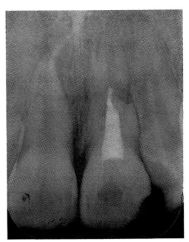

ROOT FRACTURE

## General prognosis

Two major factors can predict prognosis for pulpal healing after root fracture: the stage of root development at the time of injury and dislocation of the coronal fragment. Figs. 4.8 and 4.9 show the risk of pulp necrosis as related to the stage of root development. Other complications, such as progressive root resorption and loss of marginal bone support are very rare.

It should be noted that, while healing by hard tissue union is optimal, interposition of connective tissue is also an acceptable healing entity. It is not presently known how the two forms of healing affect the life expectancy of root-fractured incisors.

Finally, location of the root fracture has not been shown to affect pulp survival after injury. Thus, in patients with good periodontal health, root fractures of the cervical third could be treated successfully by permanent interproximal fixation using the acid-etch technique.


## Essentials

- Take radiographs with various angulations to diagnose fracture type and location.
- Reposition the coronal fragment and use firm splinting for 3 months.
- Check for pulpal complications after 3 weeks, 6 weeks and 3 months.
- If pulp necrosis occurs, as indicated radiographically by resorption of bone at the level of the fracture, extirpate the pulp to the level of the fracture and use calcium hydroxide as an interim dressing. After hard tissue closure of the root canal at the fracture line has been achieved (usually after 6 months to 1 year), a definitive root filling with gutta percha is made.

**Prognosis**

Pulp necrosis is infrequent (approximately 25%) and is related to displacement of the coronal fragment and mature root formation. Progressive root resorption (i.e. inflammatory resorption, ankylosis) is rare.

Fig. 4.8. Pulp survival after root fracture in teeth with open apices according to type of luxation injury (after Andreasen et al. 1989).

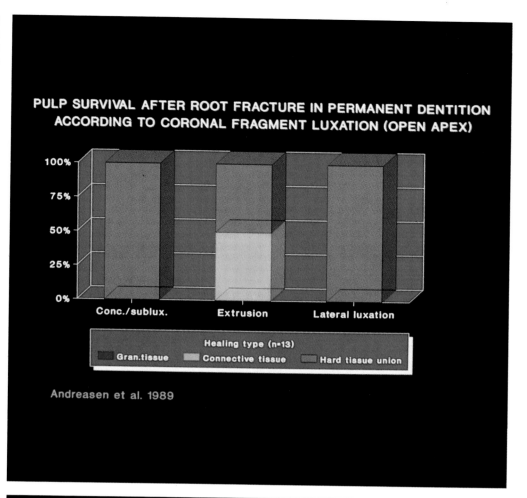

Fig. 4.9. Pulp survival after root fracture in teeth with closed apices according to type of luxation injury (after Andreasen et al. 1989).

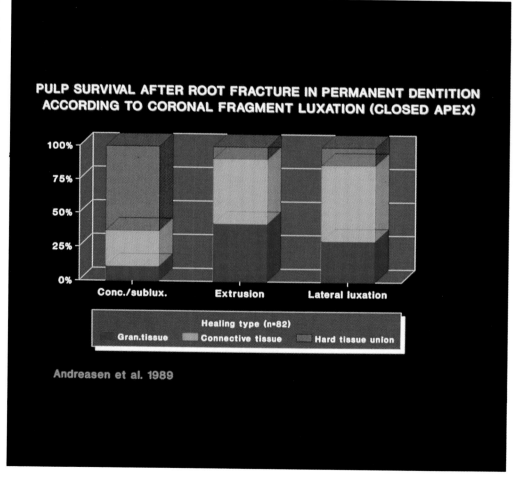

# CHAPTER 5

# Concussion and subluxation

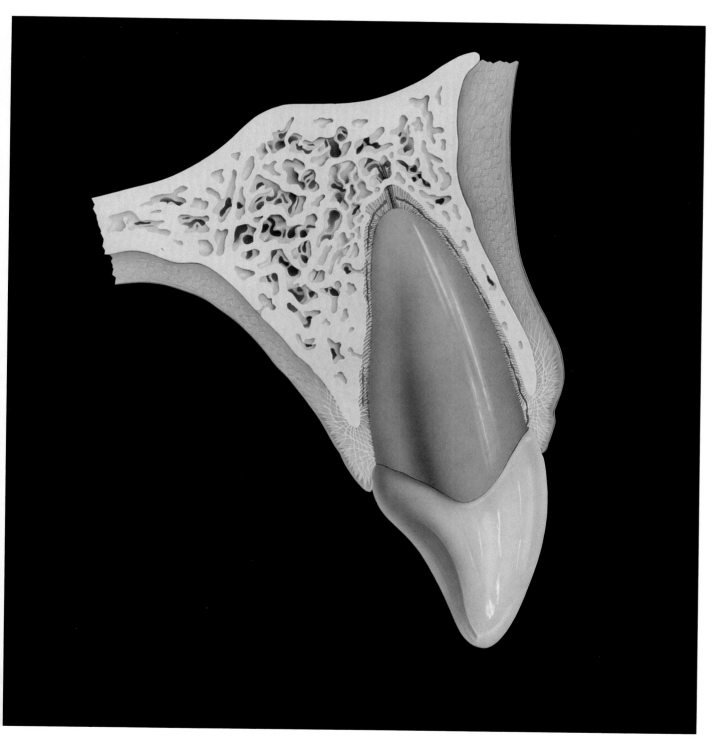

77

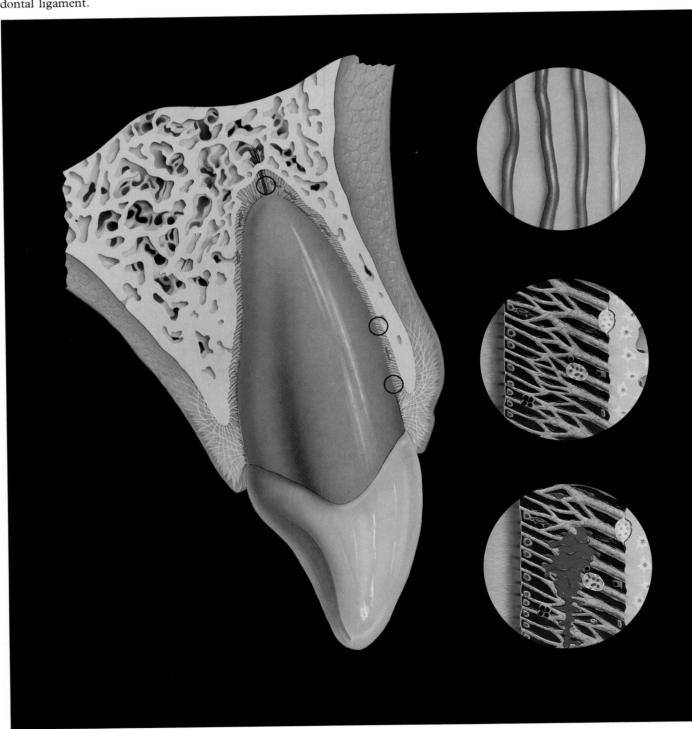

Fig. 5.2. **Mechanism of sub-luxation injury**
If the impact has greater force, periodontal ligament fibers may be torn, resulting in loosening of the injured tooth.

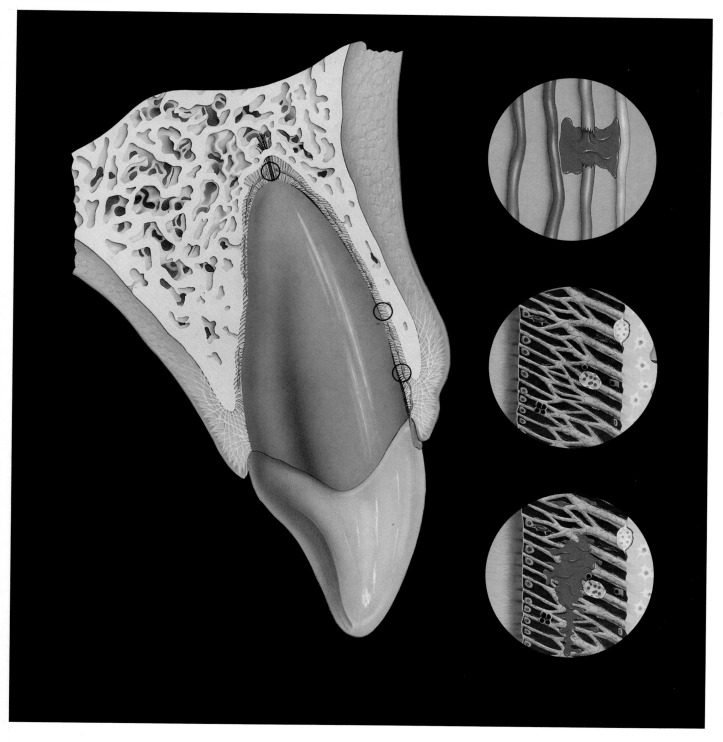

CONCUSSION AND SUBLUXATION

# Pattern of injury and diagnosis

These injuries represent minor injuries to the periodontal ligament and pulp caused by an acute impact (Fig. 5.1). In case of *concussion*, the impact can result in hemorrhage and edema within the periodontal ligament, rendering the tooth tender to percussion and mastication. However, as periodontal ligament fibers are intact, the tooth is firm in its socket and there is no bleeding from the gingival sulcus. Radiographically, there is no sign of pathology (Fig. 5.3). The neurovascular supply to the pulp is usually unaffected by the trauma, usually responding normally to electrometric sensibility testing at the time of injury (see also Appendix 3, page 160).

Greater impact to the tooth will result in *subluxation*, whereby some periodontal ligament fibers will be ruptured and the tooth loosened, but not displaced (Fig. 5.2). There is often slight bleeding from the gingival sulcus (Fig. 5.3).

## Treatment

The treatment of both types of injury consists of relief of occlusal interferences (Fig. 5.4) and ordination of a soft diet for approximately 2 weeks. Splinting of the involved teeth is not necessary, but might be desired for the comfort of the patient. If performed,

Fig. 5.3. **Clinical and radiographic features of concussion and subluxation**
The right and left maxillary central incisors have received a blow and are tender to percussion. The right central incisor is firm in its socket (concussion). While the left central incisor is loose with bleeding from the gingival sulcus (subluxation).

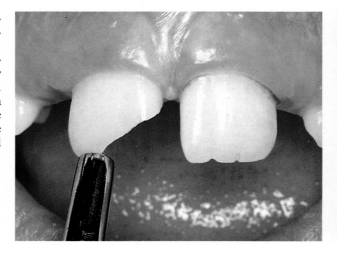 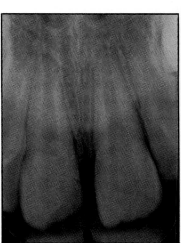

the teeth should be immobilized for not more than 2 weeks. However, fixation does not appear to promote healing.

## Follow-up procedure

Due to the slight risk of pulp necrosis, sensibility testing should be performed at the time of injury and 1 and 2 months after trauma.

## General prognosis

Due to an associated injury to the blood vessels at the root apex, pulp necrosis may occur especially in teeth with a narrow apical foramen (Figs. 5.5 and 5.7). Root resorption, however, is very rare (Figs. 5.6. and 5.8).

**Fig. 5.4. Treatment of injury**
Relief of occlusal interference by selective grinding of opposing teeth is the treatment of choice.

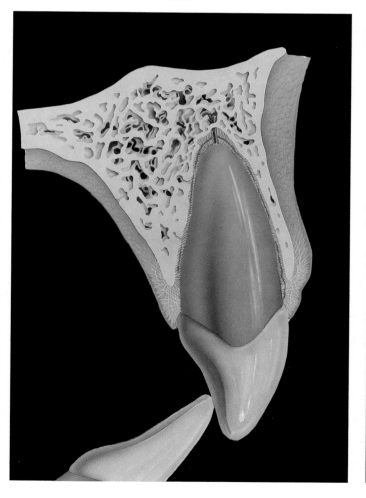
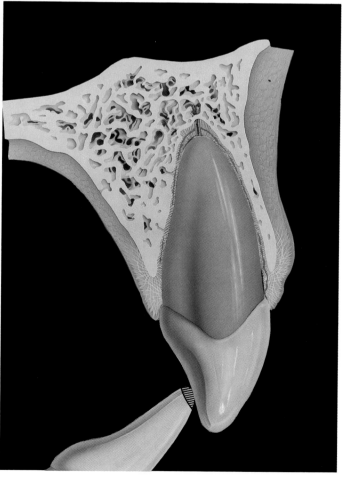

81

Fig. 5.5. **Pulp survival after concussion** (after Andreasen & Vestergaard Pedersen 1985).

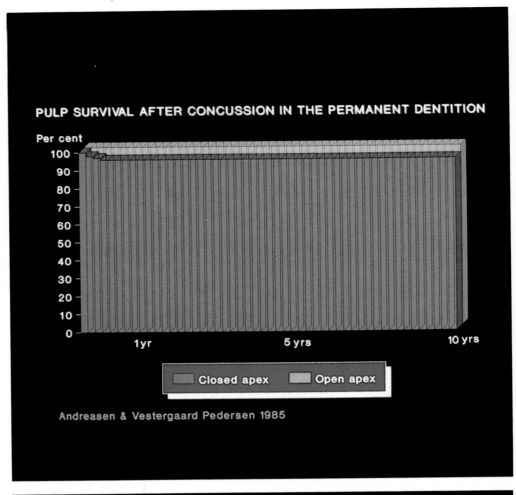

Fig. 5.6. **Periodontal healing after concussion** (after Andreasen & Vestergaard Pedersen 1985).

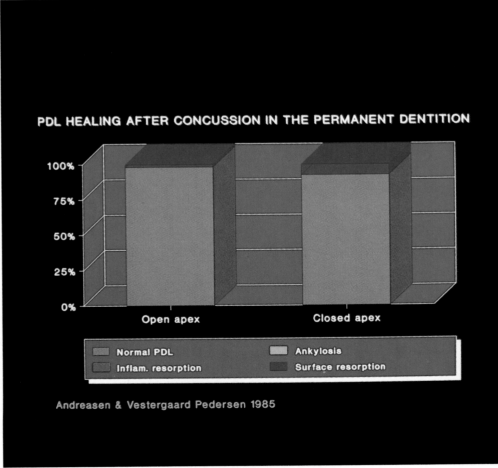

82

Fig. 5.7. **Pulp survival after subluxation** (after Andreasen & Vestergaard Pedersen 1985).

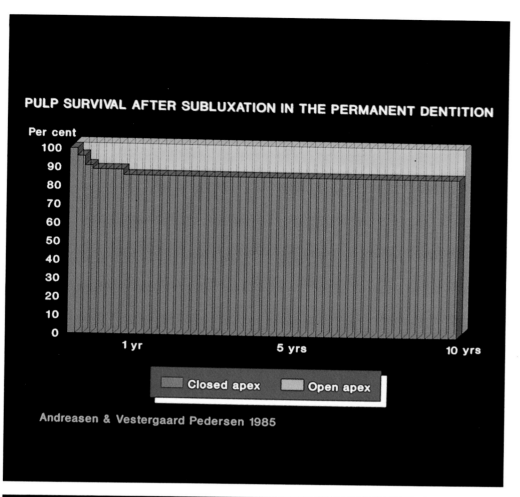

Fig. 5.8. **Periodontal healing after subluxation** (after Andreasen & Vestergaard Pedersen 1985).

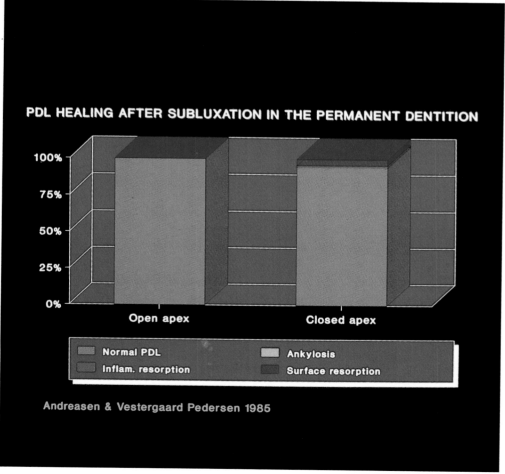

83

## Essentials

- A *concussed* tooth is tender to percussion due to edema and hemorrhage in the PDL.
- A *subluxated* tooth is tender to percussion and also abnormally loose, due to rupture of PDL fibers.

Treatment consists of:

- Occlusal relief (e.g. by selective grinding of opposing teeth) and a soft diet.
- Immobilization of the injured teeth may be appropriate for patient comfort. However, splinting does not appear to promote healing. The fixation period is 2 weeks.

## Prognosis

There is only a minimal risk of pulp necrosis and even less risk of progressive root resorption.

# Extrusion and lateral luxation

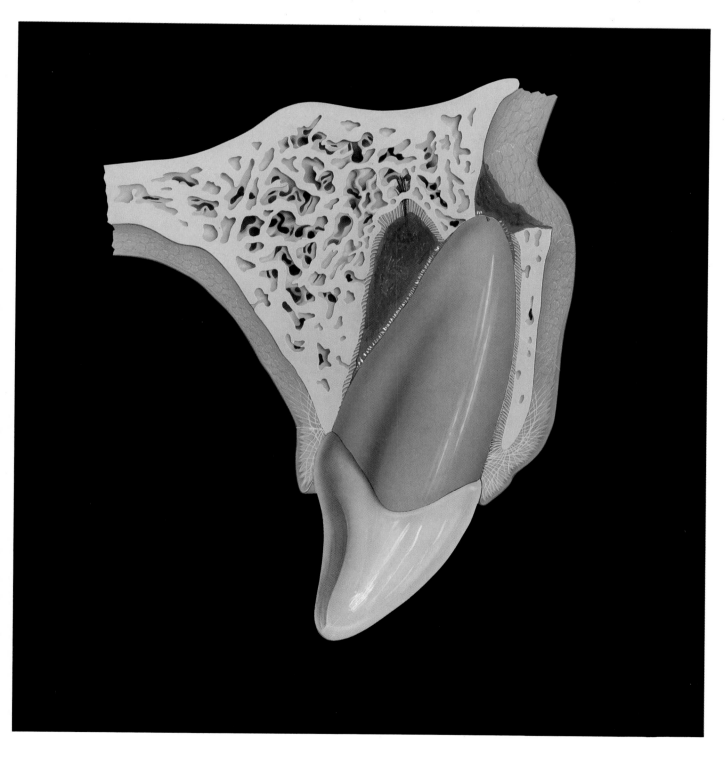

EXTRUSION AND LATERAL LUXATION

Fig. 6.1. **Pathogenesis of extrusive luxation**
Oblique forces displace the tooth out of its socket. Only the gingival fibers palatally prevent the tooth from being avulsed. Both the PDL and the neurovascular supply to the pulp is severed.

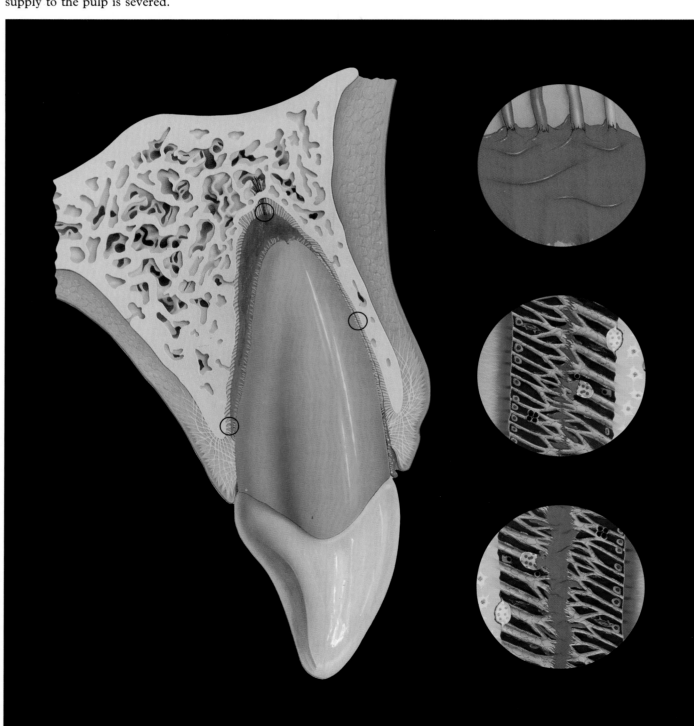

**Fig. 6.2. Pathogenesis of lateral luxation**
Horizontal forces displace the crown palatally and the apex labially. Apart from severance of the PDL and the neurovascular supply to the pulp, compression of the PDL is found on the palatal aspect of the root.

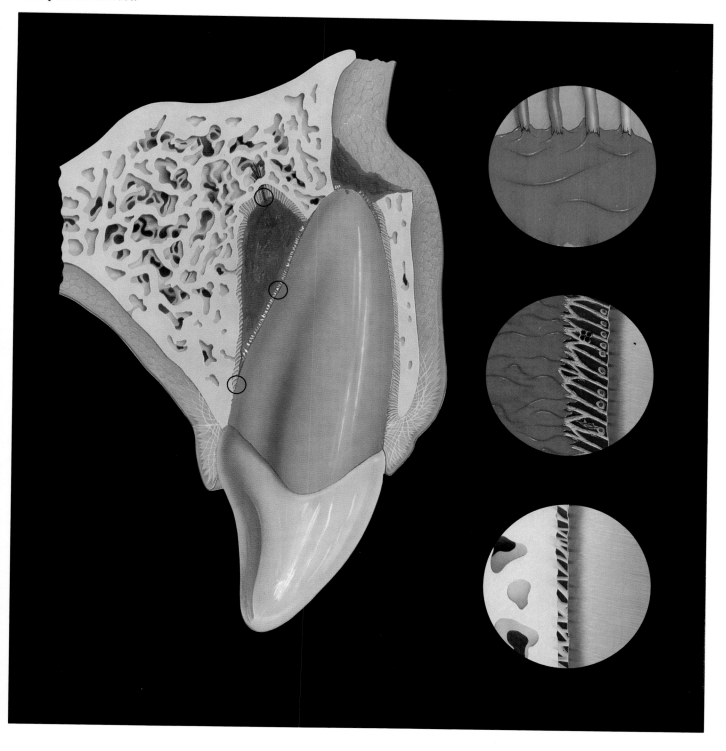

87

Fig. 6.3. **Clinical and radiographic features of extrusive luxation**
The bisecting angle radiographic technique is more useful than an occlusal exposure in revealing displacement.

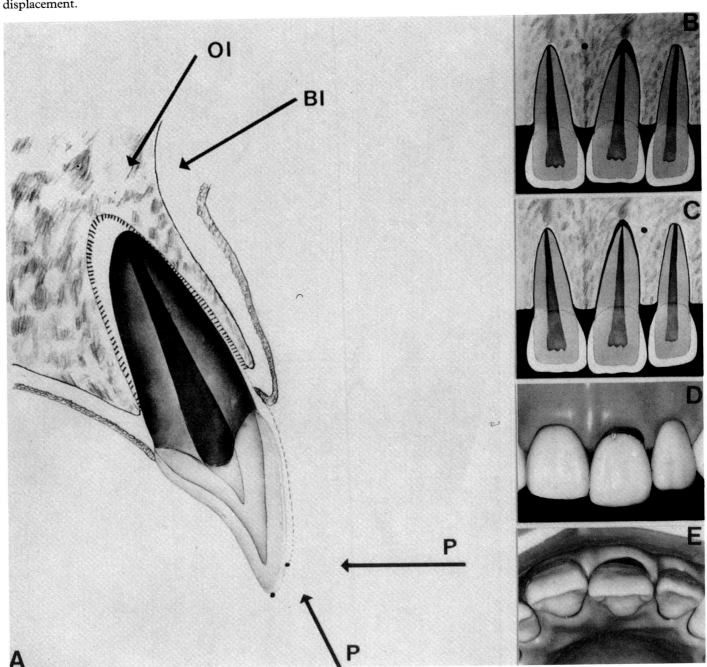

Fig. 6.4. **Clinical and radiographic features of lateral luxation**
The occlusal radiographic exposure or the eccentric bisecting angle exposure are more useful than an orthoradial bisecting angle in revealing displacement.

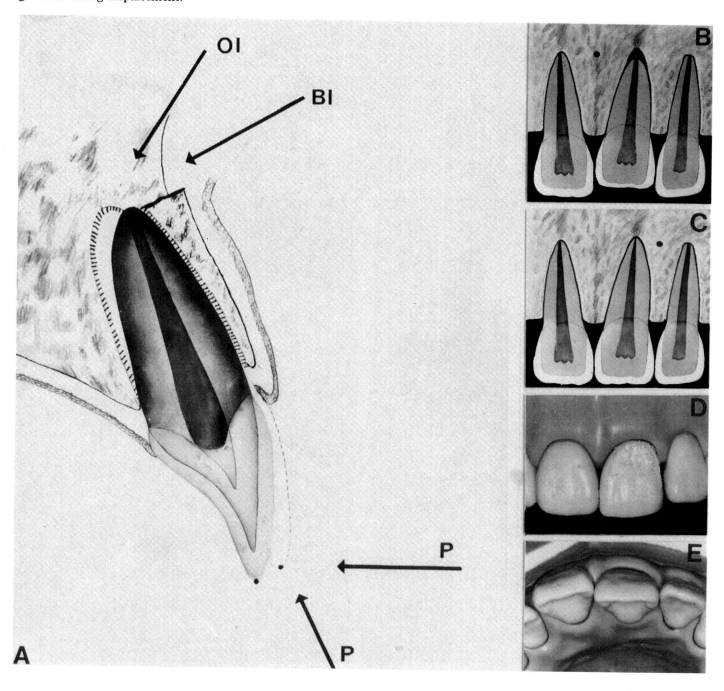

89

# Pattern of injury and diagnosis

In these two types of injury, there is a combined periodontal and pulpal injury. In the case of *extrusion*, the acute impact forces the tooth out of its socket, while the palatal periodontal ligament fibers prevent total avulsion (Fig. 6.1). In *lateral luxation*, a horizontal impact forces the crown palatally and the apex labially. Both movements result in contusion or fracture of the alveolar socket walls. Lateral luxation thus creates a complex of compression and rupture zones in the periodontal ligament, pulp and bone (Fig. 6.2).

Clinically, the *extruded* tooth is displaced axially out of its socket and is extremely loose, being held in place by a few intact

Fig. 6.5. Treatment principles of extrusive luxation: repositioning and splinting

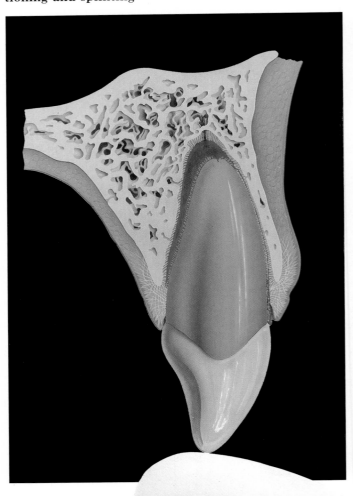
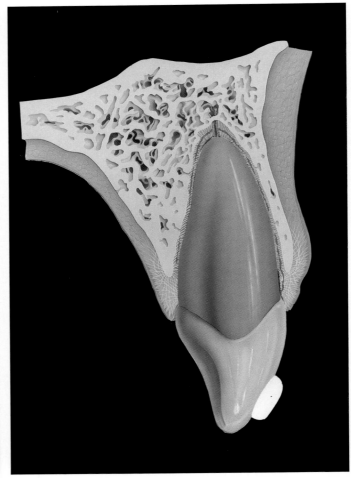

gingival fibers palatally. Radiographically, a periapical bisecting angle exposure is more useful than an occlusal exposure (Fig. 6.3).

Clinically, the crown of the *laterally luxated tooth* is usually displaced horizontally, with the tooth locked firmly in the new position, thereby eliciting a high metallic percussion (ankylosis) tone (see also Appendix 3, page 160). Radiographic demonstration is entirely dependent upon angulation of the central beam. Thus, a standard orthoradial periapical bisecting angle technique will usually fail to disclose displacement, due to overlapping of the root of the tooth and bone; whereas a more occlusally or eccentrically oriented exposure will tend to come between the root of the tooth and the empty socket, thus revealing the true nature of the injury (Fig. 6.4).

Healing subsequent to *extrusion* depends upon whether repositioning has been optimal. If so, pulpal revascularization and healing will take place as described for replantation. If repositioning has been less than optimal, revascularization will be retarded both in the pulp and periodontal ligament. In a tooth with immature root formation, arrested root development can be expected due to irreversible damage to the Hertwig's epithelial root sheath.

Healing after *lateral luxation* is entirely dependent upon the complex healing pattern resulting from the combined pulpal and periodontal injuries. Thus, the final outcome can range from pulpal and periodontal regeneration/repair to infected pulp necrosis and external root resorption and loss of gingival attachment. The exact circumstances leading to these complications have not yet been identified.

## Treatment

Treatment consists of atraumatic repositioning and fixation which prevents excessive movement during the healing period. The value of antibiotic therapy is thus far unknown.

Repositioning of *extruded* incisors is achieved by a slow and steady apical pressure which gradually displaces the coagulum formed between the root apex and floor of the socket as the tooth is moved apically. Thereafter, an acid-etch splint is applied and maintained for 2 – 3 weeks (Figs. 6.5 and 6.6).

*Laterally luxated* incisors should be repositioned with as little force as possible (Figs. 6.7 and 6.8). Thus, careful planning is decisive for the repositioning sequence. The general principles follow that of repositioning of tooth segments after fracture of the alveolar process; that is, freeing the apical lock in the cortical labial bone plate (see Chapter 9). This can be achieved either by digital pressure or surgically, with forceps, whereafter the tooth is repositioned apically. Digital pressure is presumably the gentlest 91

**Fig. 6.6. Diagnosis and treatment of extrusive luxation**
This 17-year-old man has extruded the left central incisor and avulsed the lateral incisor, which could not be retrieved.

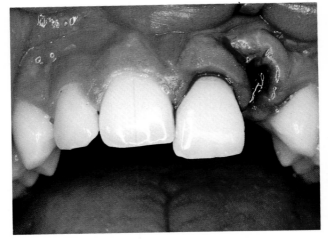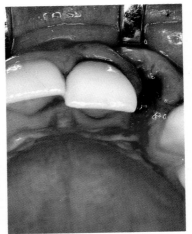

**Mobility and percussion test**
The tooth is very mobile and can be moved in horizontal and axial direction. The percussion test reveals slight tenderness and there is a dull percussion tone.

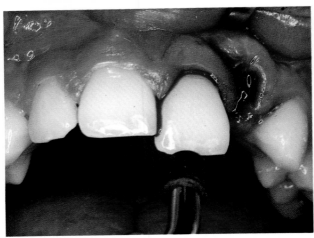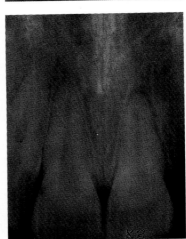

**Sensibility testing and radiographic examination**
The tooth does not respond to sensibility testing. The radiographic examination shows coronal displacement of the tooth.

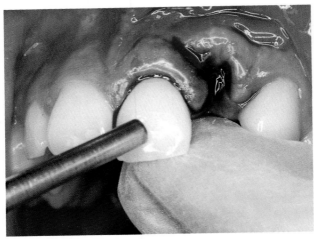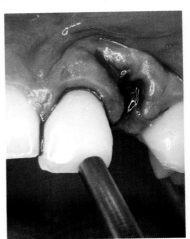

**Repositioning**
The tooth is gently pushed back into its socket. Thereafter the labial surfaces of both central incisors are etched in preparation for splinting.

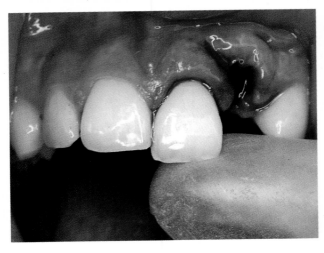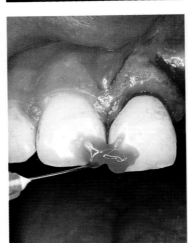

92

**Applying splinting material**
After rinsing the labial surfaces with water and drying with compressed air, the splinting material (Protemp® Espe Corp.) is applied.

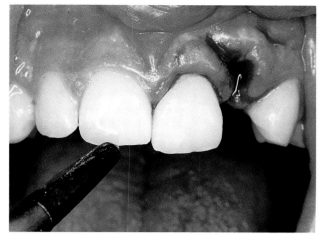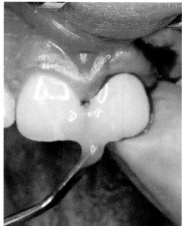

**Polishing the splint**
The surface of the splint is smoothed with abrasive discs and contact with the gingiva removed with a straight scalpel blade.

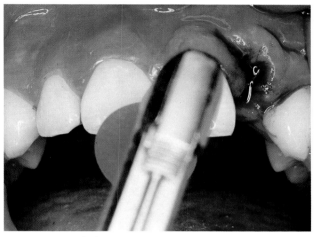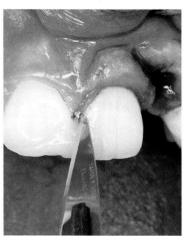

**The finished splint**
Note that the splint allows optimal oral hygiene in the gingival region which is the most likely port of entry for bacteria which may complicate periodontal and pulpal healing.

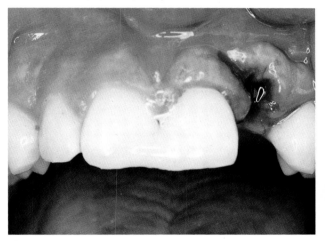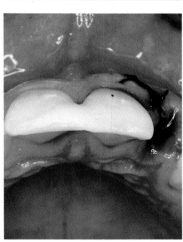

**Suturing the gingival wound**
The gingival wound is closed with interrupted silk sutures. The final radiograph shows optimal repositioning of the tooth.

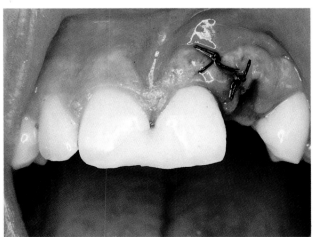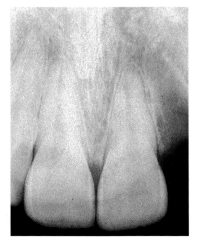

treatment. In this context, correct positioning of the clinician is essential in successful repositioning with digital pressure. Thus, if the operator stands slightly behind the patient, it is possible to palpate the displaced apex in the sulcular fold and with steady pressure force it free of its bony lock. Often a click will be heard as the apex is freed. It is then possible to reposition the tooth. An acid-etch splint is then applied for 3 weeks (Fig. 6.8).

With respect to repositioning of *extruded* teeth, it is not necessary to administer a local anesthetic as repositioning can be achieved rather easily with minimum discomfort to the patient. However, it is recommended that local anesthetic be used prior to repositioning of *laterally luxated* incisors. This can be accomplished by using an infraorbital regional block on the affected side.

At the time of repositioning, the laterally luxated incisor might appear firm in its position and fixation seem unnecessary. However, it should be considered that temporary breakdown of the marginal bone may occur within 2-4 weeks, resulting in looseness of the luxated tooth and thus requiring fixation for patient comfort (see later).

Fig. 6.7. **Treatment principles for lateral luxation: repositioning and splinting**

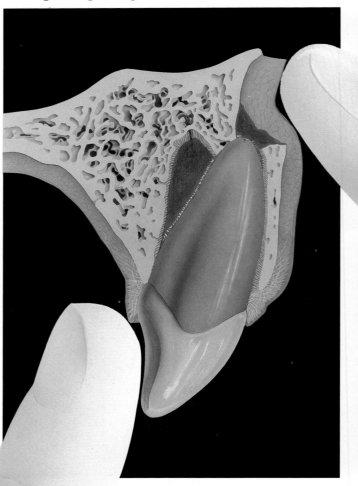 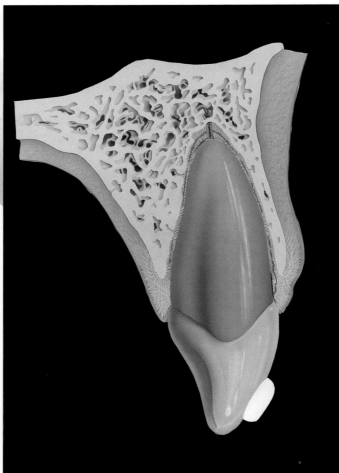

94

## Fig. 6.8. Diagnosis and treatment of lateral luxation

This 23-year-old man suffered a lateral luxation of the right central incisor.

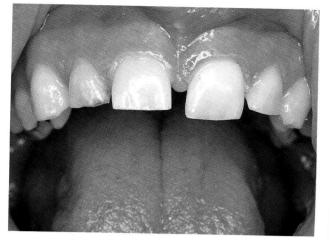

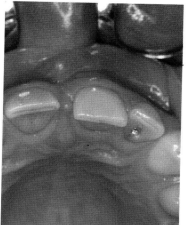

### Percussion test

Percussion of the injured tooth will reveal a high metallic sound.

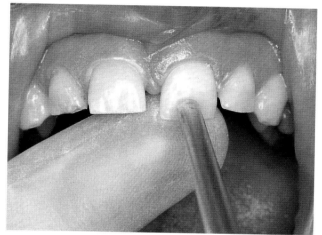

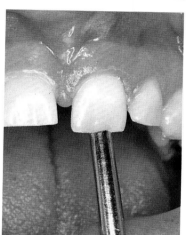

### Mobility and sensibility testing

Mobility testing, using either digital pressure or alternating pressure of two instrument handles facially and orally, reveals no mobility of the injured tooth. There is no response to pulpal sensibility testing.

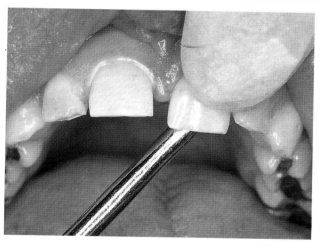

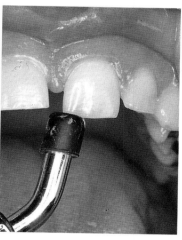

### Radiographic examination

A steep occlusal radiographic exposure reveals, as expected, more displacement than the bisecting angle technique. A lateral radiograph reveals the associated fracture of the labial bone plate (arrow).

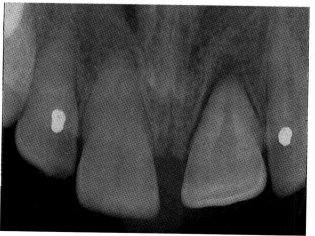

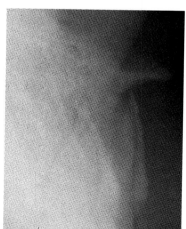

EXTRUSION AND LATERAL LUXATION

### Anesthesia
An infraorbital regional block is placed and supplemented with anesthesia of the nasopalatinal nerve.

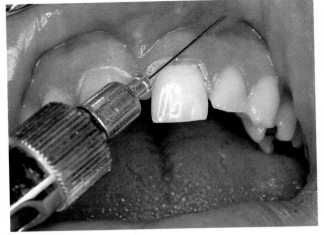 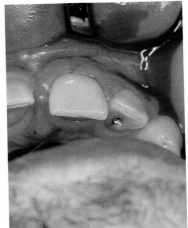

### Repositioning
The tooth is repositioned initially by forcing the displaced apex past the labial bone lock and thereby disengaging the root. Thereafter, axial pressure apically will bring the tooth back to its original position. It should be remembered that the palatal aspect of the marginal bone has also been displaced at the time of impact. This must be repositioned with digital pressure to ensure optimal periodontal healing.

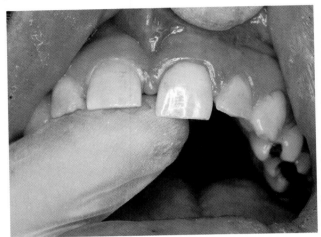 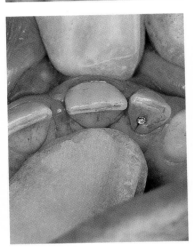

### Verifying repositioning and splinting with the acid-etch technique
Occlusion is checked and a radiograph taken to verify adequate repositioning. The incisal one-third of the labial aspect of the injured and adjacent teeth are acid-etched (30 seconds) with phosphoric acid gel.

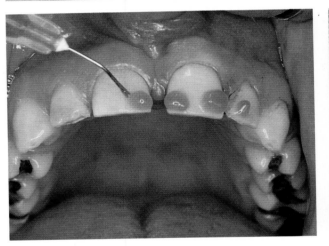 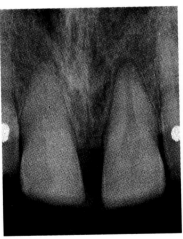

### Preparing the splinting material
The etchant is removed with a 20 seconds water spray. The labial enamel is dried with compressed air, revealing the mat, etched surface.

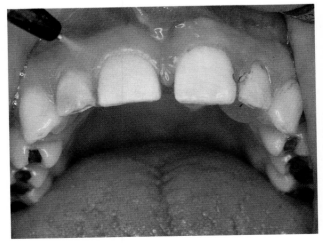 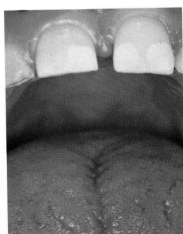

96

## Applying the splinting material

A temporary crown and bridge material (e.g. Protemp®) is then applied. Surplus material can be removed after polymerization using a straight scalpel blade, abrasive discs or a fissure bur.

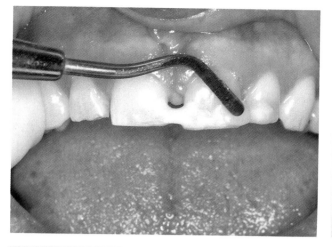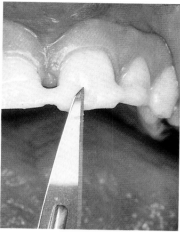

## Three weeks after injury

At this examination, a radiograph is taken to evaluate periodontal and pulpal healing. That is, neither periapical radiolucency nor breakdown of supporting marginal bone, as compared to the radiograph taken after repositioning.

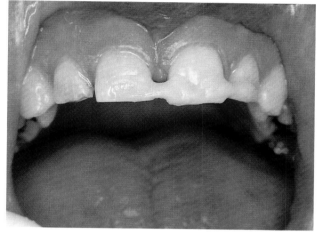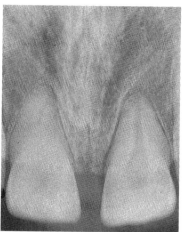

## Splint removal

The splint is removed using fissure burs, by reducing the splinting material interproximally and thereafter thinning the splint uniformly across its total span. Once thinned out, the splint can be removed using a sharp explorer.

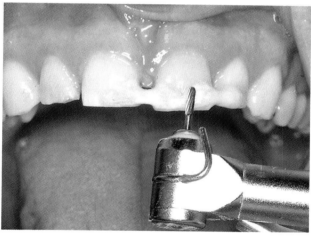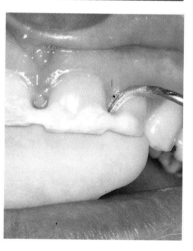

## Six months after injury

After 6 months, there is a slight sensibility reaction and normal radiographic conditions.

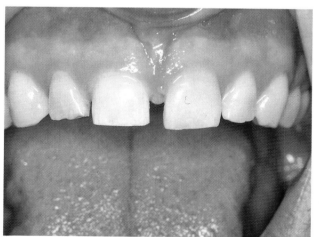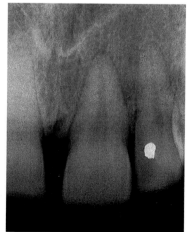

EXTRUSION AND LATERAL LUXATION

## Follow-up procedures

The splint may be removed 2 – 3 weeks after *extrusion*. Three weeks after *lateral luxation* and prior to splint removal, a radiograph is taken to ascertain healing. Due to the extent of trauma, osteoclastic activity may result in a temporary breakdown of the marginal bone, seen as a rarefaction of the marginal periodontium (Fig. 6.9). In this case, it may be necessary to maintain fixation for up to 2 months. Optimal oral hygiene is also necessary during this period. If such changes are not present, the splint may be removed after 3 weeks (see also Appendix 4, page 161).

External inflammatory root resorption may also occur, requiring immediate endodontic therapy with calcium hydroxide as an interim dressing (see page 122).

Also at this time, sensibility testing should be performed. An observation period of up to 12 months or more can pass before a positive response to pulp testing can be expected in these teeth.

## General prognosis

The prognosis for extruded and laterally luxated teeth with respect to pulpal and periodontal healing depends upon the stage of root development at the time of injury (Figs. 6.10 to 6.13).

Fig. 6.9. **Transient marginal breakdown**
In this case, temporary loss of marginal bone support is seen 3 weeks after injury, which was later followed by reformation of supporting bone.

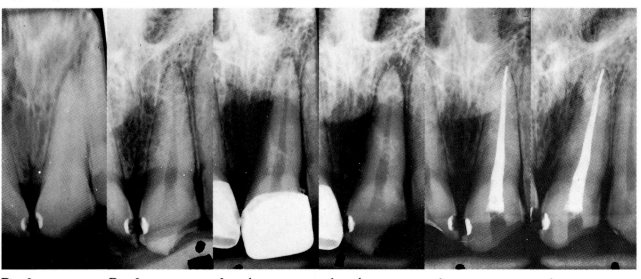

| Day 0 | Day 0 | 3 weeks | 6 weeks | 1 year | 1 year |

Fig. 6.10. **Pulpal healing after extrusive luxation** (after Andreasen & Vestergaard Pedersen 1985).

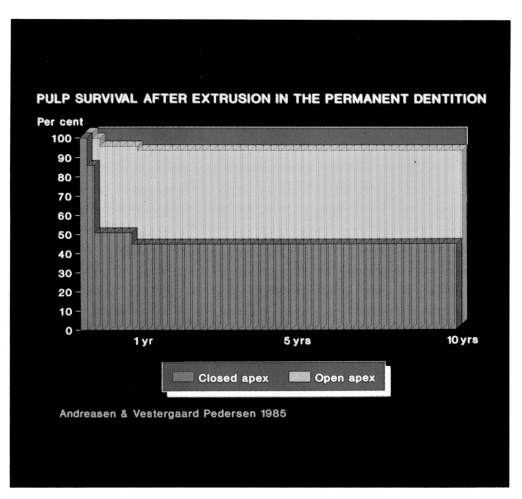

Fig. 6.11. **Periodontal healing after extrusive luxation** (after Andreasen & Vestergaard Pedersen 1985).

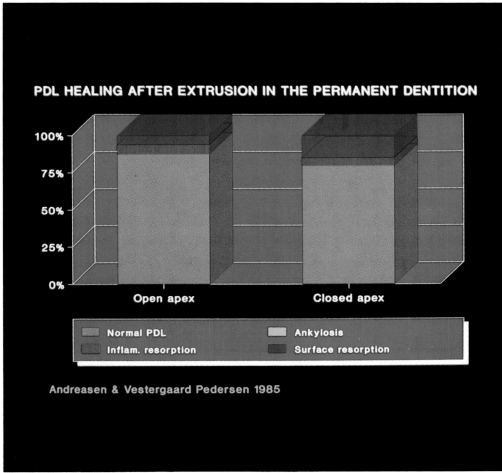

EXTRUSION AND LATERAL LUXATION

Fig. 6.12. **Pulpal healing after lateral luxation** (after Andreasen & Vestergaard Pedersen 1985).

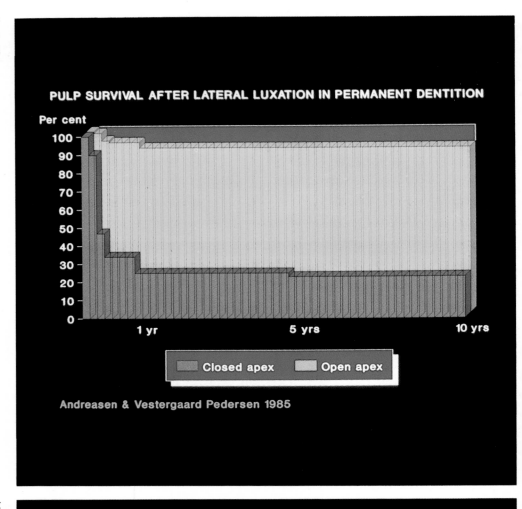

Fig. 6.13. **Periodontal healing after lateral luxation** (after Andreasen & Vestergaard Pedersen 1985).

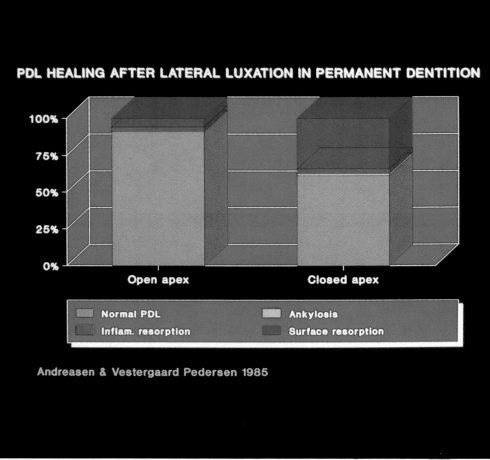

CHAPTER 6

## Essentials

- **Extrusive luxation** represents a rupture of the PDL and the pulp.
- **Lateral luxation** represents a rupture of the PDL and the pulp as well as injury to the labial and/or palatal alveolar bone plate.
- In both cases, healing includes both PDL repair and usually pulpal revascularization.

Treatment consists of:
- Atraumatic repositioning and fixation.
- In the case of lateral luxation, administration of local anesthetic is necessary prior to repositioning.
- Radiographic examination after 2-3 weeks.

If radiographic examination reveals no sign of marginal breakdown, the splint can be removed. Otherwise further controls are necessary.

If radiographic examination reveals inflammatory resorption of the bone and root, immediate endodontic therapy is required.

## Prognosis

There is considerable risk of pulp necrosis in both luxation categories, especially in teeth with mature root formation. Progressive root resorption is rare after extrusion (Fig. 6.11); but can occur following lateral luxation (Fig. 6.13).

101

# CHAPTER 7

# Intrusion

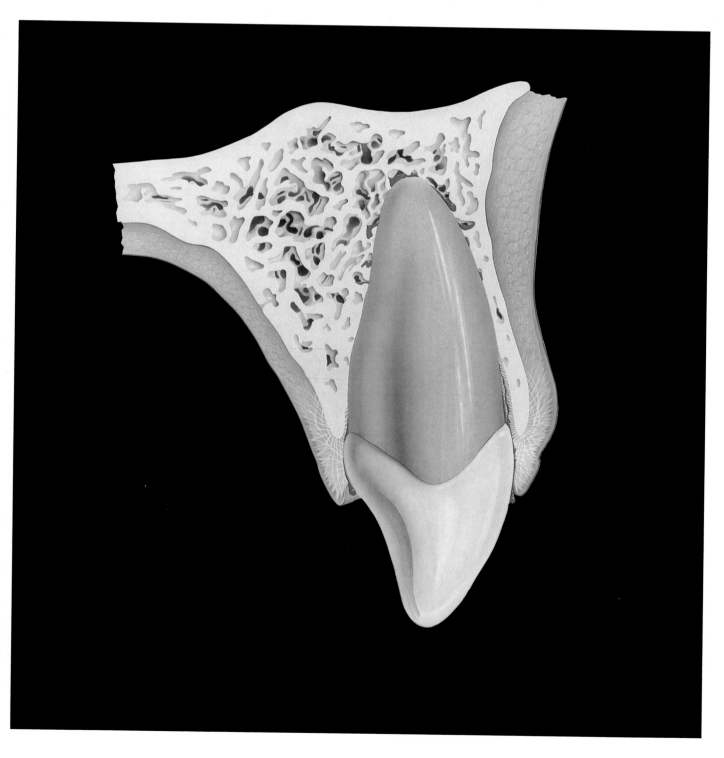

103

Fig. 7.1. **Pathogenesis of intrusion**
Axial impact leads to extensive injury to the pulp and periodontium.

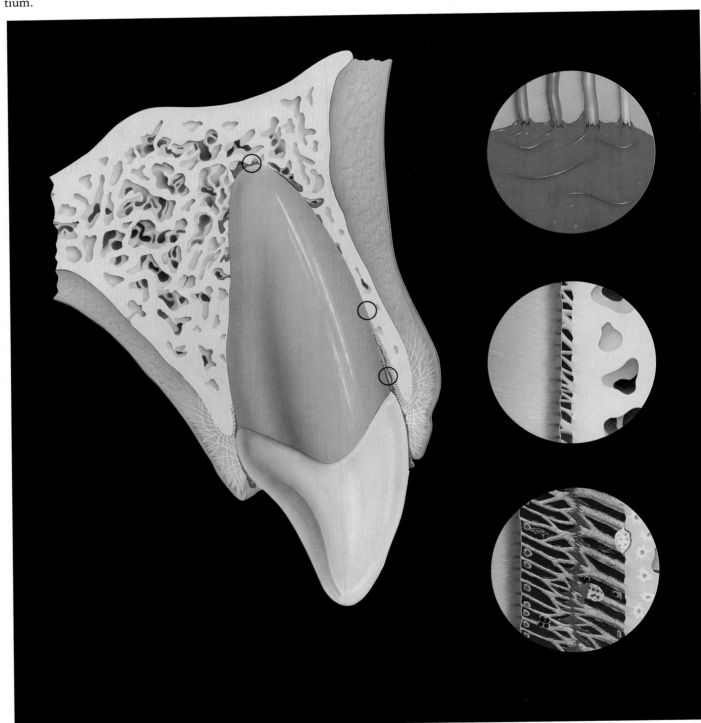

# Pattern of injury and diagnosis

In this type of injury, maximum damage has occurred to pulp and all supporting structures, as the tooth has been driven into the alveolar process due to an axially directed impact (Fig. 7.1). The resulting damage is dependent upon the age of the patient.

In the adult dentition, diagnosis of intrusive luxation is primarily dependent upon the difference in incisal height of the affected and adjacent non-affected teeth (Fig. 7.2). In the mixed dentition, diagnosis is more difficult, as the intrusion can mimic a tooth under eruption. The percussion test, however, will reveal whether the tooth in question is under eruption (a dull tone) or locked into bone (a high metallic tone, pathognomonic for intrusion or lateral luxation, see Appendix 3, page 160) (Fig. 7.3).

Healing after intrusion is usually complicated, as the extensive injury to the PDL can lead to progressive external root resorption (ankylosis). Likewise, damage to the pulp bears with it the risk of inflammatory resorption. Treatment should, therefore, be directed towards eliminating or reducing the extent of both of these healing complications.

**Fig. 7.2. Intrusion of a tooth with completed root formation**
The difference in the level of the incisal edge, as well as the apical shift of the cemento-enamel junction indicates intrusion.

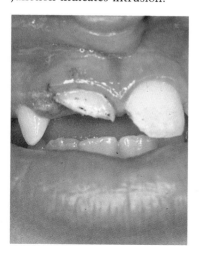
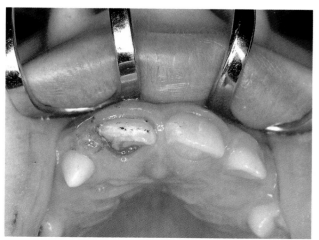
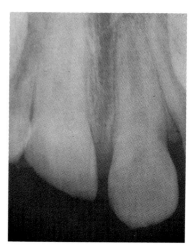

105

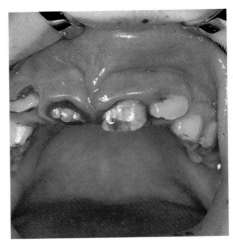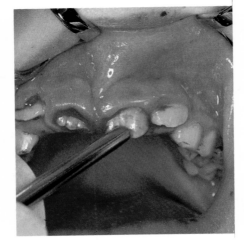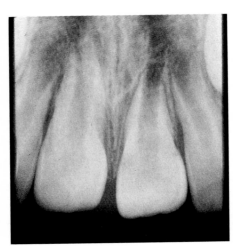

Fig. 7.3. Intrusion of a tooth with incomplete root formation
The semi-erupted position of the tooth leaves doubt about whether the tooth is under eruption or intruded from a more coronal position. A high percussion (ankylosis) tone reveals the intrusion.

Fig. 7.4. Treatment principles of intrusions: spontaneous eruption or orthodontic extrusion

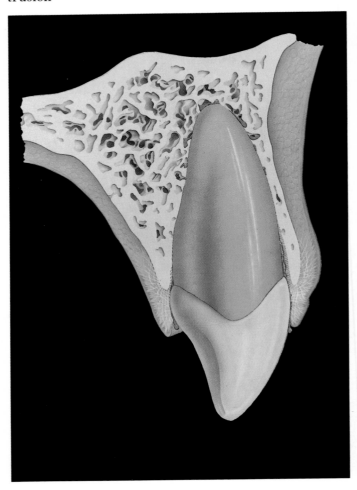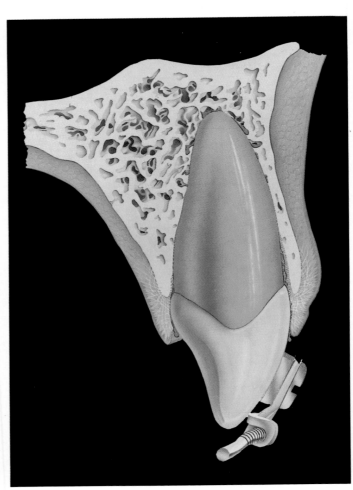

106

## Treatment

Treatment principles for intruded permanent incisors are entirely dependent upon the stage of root development (Figs. 7.4 and 7.5). In the case of immature root formation, spontaneous re-eruption can be anticipated. During this process, the crushed cervical bone is usually repaired. As spontaneous re-eruption can occur over a period of several months, it is of utmost importance that pulpal healing is constantly monitored.

In cases where a periapical radiolucency or inflammatory root resorption develop, it is essential that the infected pulp be extirpated as soon as the healing complication is diagnosed and the root canal dressed with calcium hydroxide paste. It should be remembered that pulp necrosis is a very frequent finding after intrusion, irrespective of stage of root development.

**Fig. 7.5. Spontaneous eruption of two intruded incisors**
Clinical and radiographic condition in a 7-year-old girl after an axial impact.

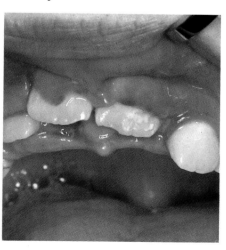

**Initial eruption**
Condition 6 weeks later, after onset of eruption.

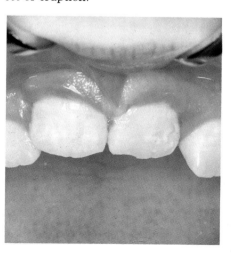

**Follow-up, 1 year after injury**
Eruption is complete.

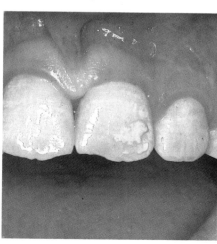

## Fig. 7.6. Orthodontic extrusion of an intruded incisor

Clinical and radiographic condition in an 22-year-old woman after an axial impact.

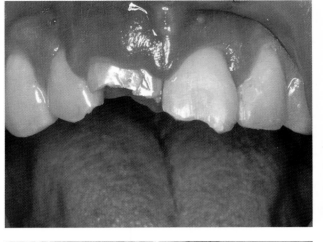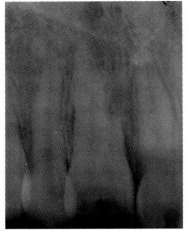

### Covering exposed dentin

The exposed dentin of both central incisors is covered with a hard-setting calcium hydroxide cement (e.g. Dycal®).

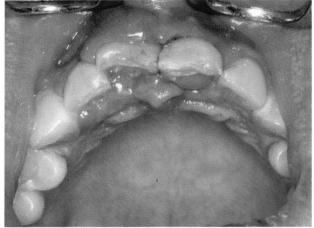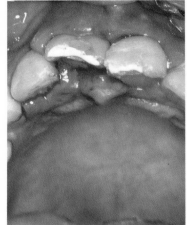

### Applying orthodontic traction

A 0.5 mm thick semi-rigid orthodontic wire is bent to follow the curvature of the dental arch, including two adjacent teeth on either side of the intruded incisor. The orthodontic wire is fastened to the adjacent teeth using an acid-etch technique. In the area where elastic traction is exerted, a coil spring (e.g. 0.228 x 0.901, Elgiloy) is placed in order to prevent slippage of the elastic.

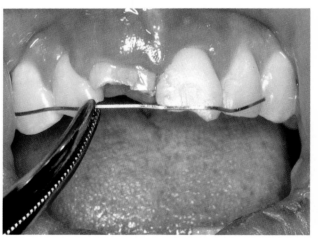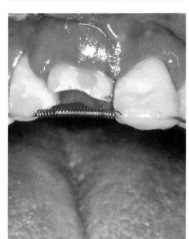

### Placing the bracket

A bracket is placed on the labial surface and the fractured incisal edge is covered with a temporary crown and bridge material.

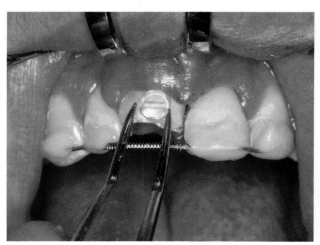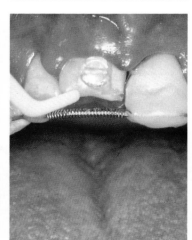

### Orthodontic traction

Elastic traction of 70 – 100 grams is activated. The direction of traction should extrude the tooth out of its socket in a purely axial direction.

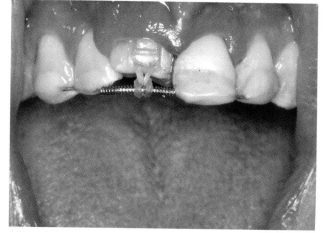
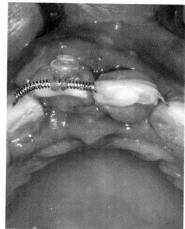

### Extrusion initiated

After approximately 10 days, osteoclastic activity around the intruded tooth has usually resulted in loosening and extrusion can then occur. If extrusion has not yet begun after 10 days, a local anesthetic is administered and the tooth is luxated slightly with a forceps. After 2 – 3 weeks, a rubber dam is applied, the pulp extirpated and the root canal is filled with calcium hydroxide paste.

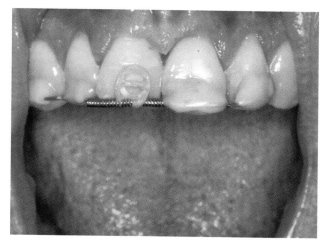
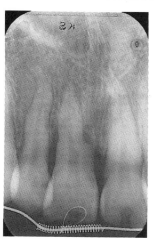

### Extrusion complete

After 4 weeks, the intruded tooth is extruded to its original position and the tooth retained in its new position for 2-4 weeks. Thereafter, the orthodontic appliance can be removed.

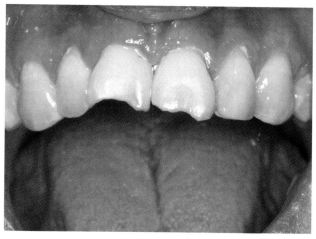
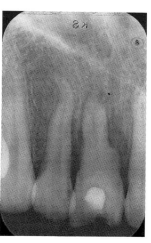

### Crown restoration

The fractured crowns are restored with composite resin.

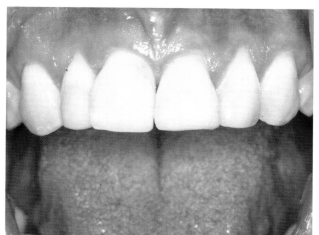
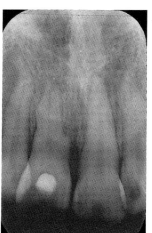

In the case of completed root development, spontaneous re-eruption is unpredictable and orthodontic extrusion is therefore indicated (Fig. 7.6). Extrusion should be accomplished over a period of 2 – 3 weeks in order to permit endodontic therapy prior to the radiographic appearance of inflammatory root resorption. As pulp necrosis following intrusion of mature teeth has been found with nearly 100% frequency, prophylactic pulp extirpation is indicated.

## Follow-up procedures

Continuous clinical and radiographic monitoring is necessary following this trauma entity as pulpal and periodontal healing complications are so frequent.

Fig. 7.7. **Pulp survival after intrusion** (after Andreasen & Vestergaard Pedersen 1985).

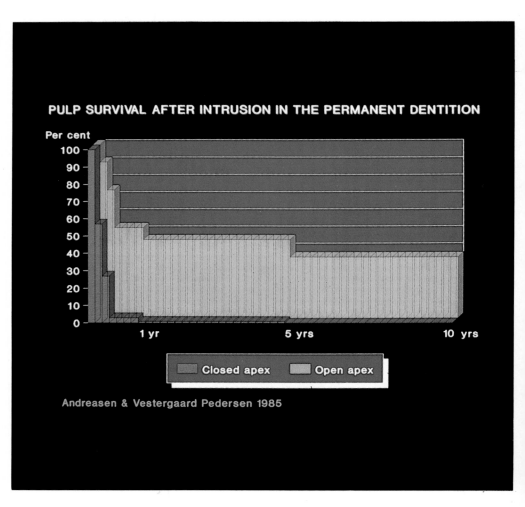

110

## General prognosis

With respect to pulp survival, only teeth with immature root formation have been shown to demonstrate pulp survival following intrusion (Fig. 7.7). With respect to periodontal healing, there is a high risk of root resorption (58% for teeth with immature root formation and 70% for teeth with mature root formation) (Fig. 7.8). Moreover, some teeth have been found to demonstrate ankylosis as late as 5 years following injury, therefore requiring extended follow-up periods.

Fig. 7.8. **Periodontal healing after intrusion** (after Andreasen & Vestergaard Pedersen 1985).

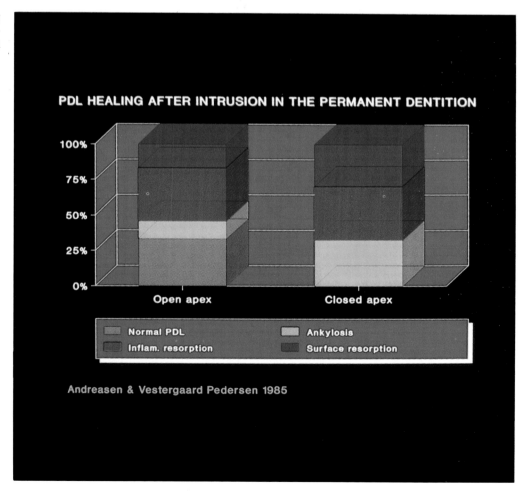

PDL HEALING AFTER INTRUSION IN THE PERMANENT DENTITION

Andreasen & Vestergaard Pedersen 1985

111

## Essentials

– Intrusion is the result of an axial, apical impact and results in extensive damage to the pulp and PDL.
– Treatment.
– **Immature root formation**
Await spontaneous re-eruption, which usually takes 2 – 4 months.

Monitor pulpal healing radiographically 3, 4 and 6 weeks after injury.
– **Mature root formation**
Await spontaneous re-eruption or extrude orthodontically over a period of 2 – 3 weeks.

Extirpate the pulp 2 weeks after injury, using calcium hydroxide paste as an interim dressing.

Root fill with a permanent gutta percha filling once periodontal healing has been established radiographically.

## Prognosis

There is a high risk of pulp necrosis and progressive root resorption, especially in teeth with mature root formation.

# Avulsion injuries

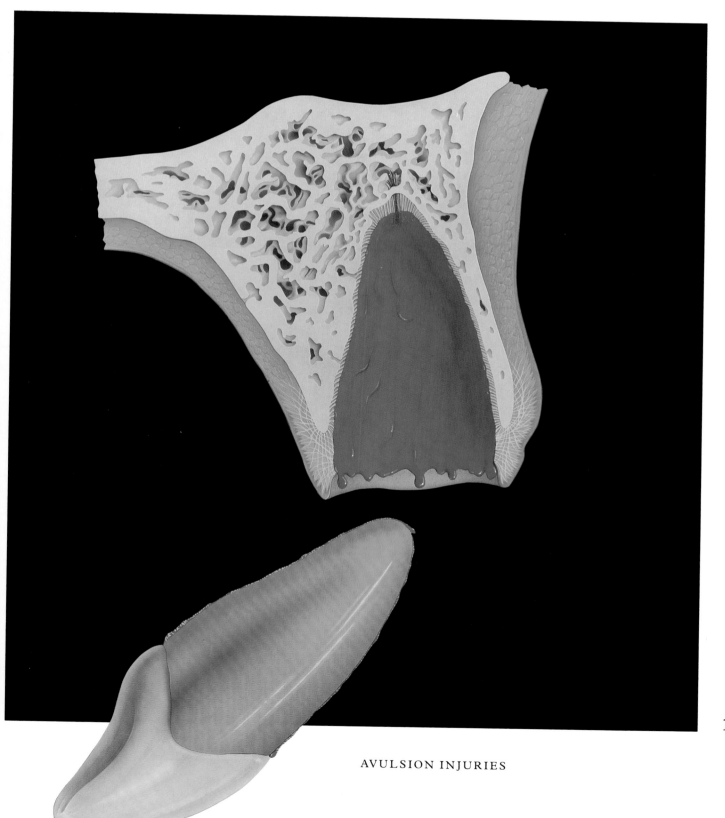

**Fig. 8.1. Mechanism of exarticulation**
Frontal impacts lead to avulsion with subsequent damage to both the pulp and periodontal ligament.

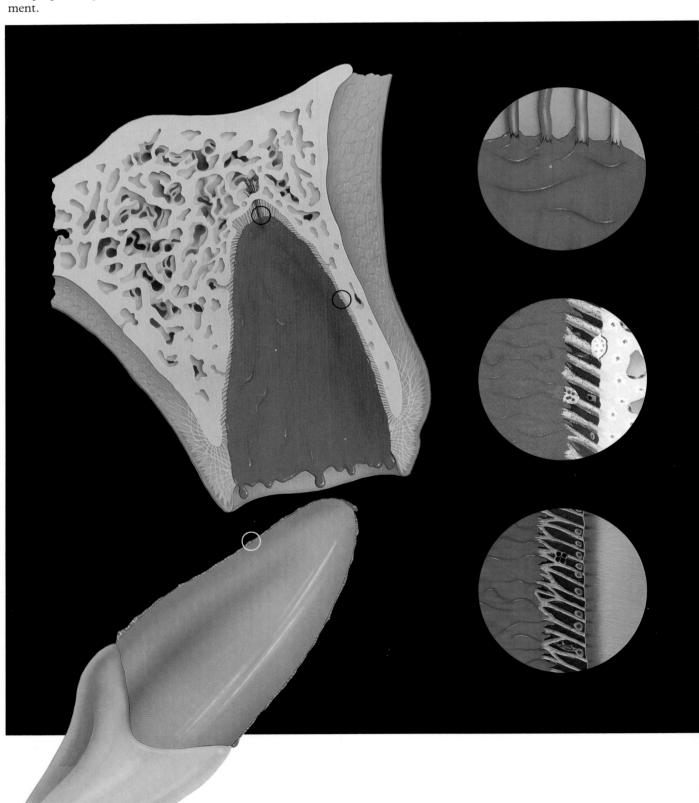

# Pattern of injury and diagnosis

Avulsion of permanent teeth is most common in the young dentition, where root development is still incomplete and the periodontium very resilient. Under these circumstances, even slight horizontal impacts may result in total dislocation of the tooth. The outcome of an eventual replantation procedure is almost entirely dependent upon the extraalveolar period and extraalveolar handling. Emphasis will, therefore, be placed on describing treatment methods which optimize healing of the periodontal ligament as well as the pulp.

The basic requirements for optimal healing are that the tooth is out of its socket for as short a period as possible, that the extraalveolar storage is in a physiologic medium and that contamination of the tooth is eliminated, reduced or controlled by antibiotics. If these conditions are met, the following healing events can be expected: Healing is accomplished by revascularization of the severed periodontal ligament, splicing of the ruptured Sharpey's fibers, formation of a new gingival attachment and, finally, revascularization and reinnervation of the pulp.

The *gingival attachment* is re-established 1 week after injury, including splicing of the ruptured gingival fibers (Fig. 8.2). Intraalveolar *periodontal ligament* revascularization is also complete and splicing of PDL fibers initiated 1 week after injury. After 2 weeks, periodontal ligament repair is so advanced that the peri-

Fig. 8.2. Healing events 2 weeks after replantation
Most of the intraalveolar periodontal fibers have healed. Pulpal revascularization has reached mid-root level.

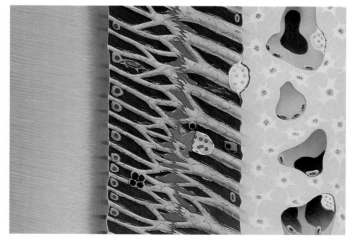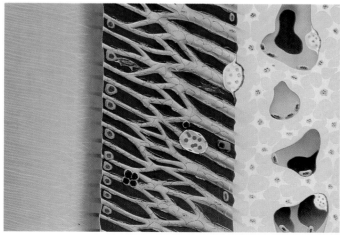

115

odontium has regained about two-thirds of its original strength (Fig. 8.2).

*Pulpal revascularization* begins 4 days after injury and proceeds at a rate of approximately 0.5 mm per day. This would imply that an entire incisor pulp in a young individual can be revascularized within 30-40 days.

In case of physical damage or bacterial contamination to the pulp or periodontal ligament, aberrations in healing will occur. Thus if there is minor damage to the innermost layer of the periodontal ligament, this site will be resorbed by macrophages and osteoclasts, resulting in a superficial excavation of the root

**Fig. 8.3. Healing with minor injury to the periodontal ligament**
The injury site is resorbed by macrophages and osteoclasts. Subsequent repair takes place with formation of new cementum and Sharpey's fibers.

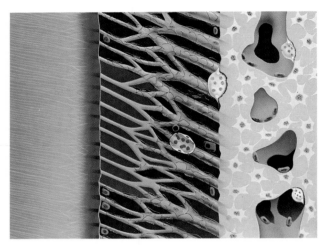

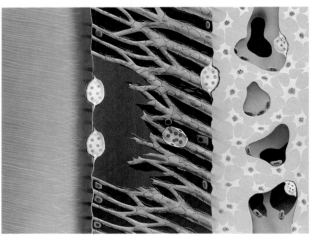

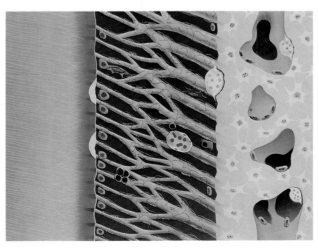

surface (Fig. 8.3). After some weeks, this resorption cavity will be repaired by new cementum and Sharpey's fibers.

In the event that the initial resorption cavity has penetrated cementum and reached the dentinal tubules, toxins from an eventual infection in the root canal or dentinal tubules can be transmitted via the exposed tubules to the root surface (Fig. 8.4). This event will lead to a continuation of the osteoclastic process and progressive resorption of the root surface, ultimately perforating to the root canal.

On the other hand, if infection in the root canal and the dentinal tubules is eliminated by endodontic therapy, osteoclastic activity

**Fig. 8.4. Healing with moderate injury to the periodontal ligament and associated infection in the pulp and/or dentinal tubules**
The initial injury to the root surface triggers a macrophage and osteoclast attack on the root surface. If the resorption cavity exposes infected tubules which can transmit bacterial toxins, the resorptive process is accelerated and granulation tissue ultimately invades the root canal.

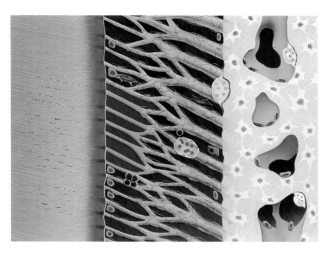

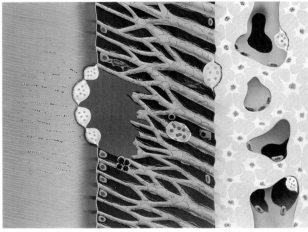

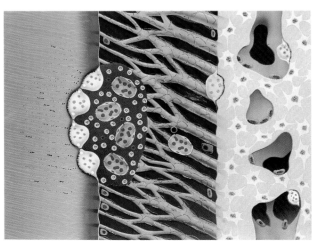

117

is arrested and healing with new cementum and Sharpey's fibers will take place.

In case of moderate to extensive damage to the innermost layer of the periodontal ligament, competitive healing processes will occur, whereby cells from the adjacent intact periodontal ligament will attempt to invade and heal the injury site; just as cells from the opposing alveolar bone will also attempt to fill out the traumatized region with new bone (Fig. 8.5). After approximately 2 weeks, bony invasion can create an ankylosis, the fate of which depends upon the extent of damage to the periodontal ligament and whether there is any functional movement of the injured

Fig. 8.5. **Healing after extensive injury to the periodontal ligament**
Ankylosis is formed because healing occurs almost exclusively by cells from the alveolar wall.

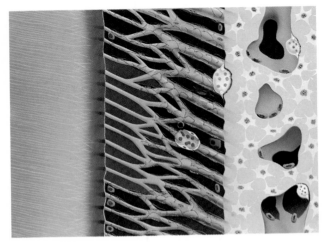

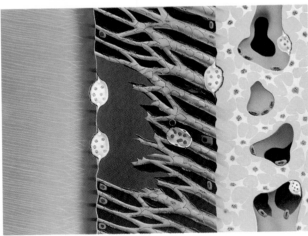

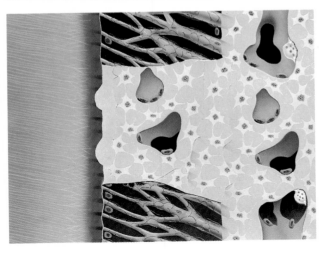

118

tooth during the healing period. If there is only minimal injury to the periodontal ligament and the tooth has not been splinted, function will stimulate osteoclastic removal of the bony bridge (i.e. transient ankylosis).

In the event of more extensive damage, and thereby a larger ankylosis site, functional stimulation will not be able to remove the ankylosis. In this case, ankylosis will be permanent (Fig. 8.5). A gradual, progressive resorption of the tooth can be expected due to the inherent remodelling of bone. This process is very active in children, whereby survival of the injured tooth can be limited to only a few years; whereas, in adults, replacement resorption is significantly slower, allowing the affected tooth to survive 10 – and sometimes even 20 – years or more.

If, during pulpal revascularization, bacteria gain access to the the ischemic pulp tissue, either via a gap in the periodontal ligament, the blood stream (anachoresis) or dentinal tubules, as after crown fracture, the revascularization process will stop and a zone of inflammation, demarcated by leucocytes, will be established. This leucocyte zone will separate the infected, ischemic pulp from the invading healing tissue. If there has also been a concomitant injury to the periodontal ligament, progressive external inflammatory root resorption will result.

## Treatment

With respect to treatment of the avulsed tooth, storage conditions and the length of the storage period are of utmost importance for successful healing. To date, the following storage media have been shown to permit both periodontal and pulpal healing: physiologic saline, blood, tissue culture media, milk and saliva. A feature common to all of these media is their relative osmotic balance with pulp and periodontal tissues. Avulsed teeth can thus be maintained for hours and in certain media (e.g. tissue culture media) even days or weeks before damage to these tissues occurs.

In the case of saliva, however, the extraalveolar period should be limited to a maximum of 2 hours due to the slight hypotonic nature of the media. Moreover, bacteria present in saliva can also have a detrimental effect on later healing.

Cleansing procedures of the root surface also influence healing. Thus, thorough rinsing of the root surface including around the apical foramen with saline should precede replantation in order to remove foreign bodies and bacteria which will stimulate an inflammatory response.

To optimize healing, the alveolus should also be flushed with saline to remove the coagulum. Recent investigations suggest that the presence of a coagulum in the socket at the time of replantation can enhance ankylosis.

119

Once the root surface and alveolus have been flushed with saline, the tooth can be replanted. This is accomplished using a minimum of pressure, being careful not to further damage the periodontal ligament and pulp. If any resistance is met, the tooth should be placed in saline and the socket visually inspected for possible fractures. Fracture of the socket wall is the most common source of difficulty in replanting avulsed teeth. The fractured bone can usually be repositioned by inserting a flat instrument (e.g. a straight elevator) and remodelling the alveolus. Replantation can then be completed. After repositioning of the tooth, a slightly flexible splint should be applied, such as an acid-etch retained splint of temporary crown and bridge material (e.g. Protemp®, Espe Co.). Unless other injuries require longer splinting periods (e.g. alveolar fracture), the splint should be removed after 7 days to allow some functional movement of the replant in order to reduce or eliminate the risk of ankylosis.

In teeth with complete root formation (i.e. the diameter of the apical foramen is less than 1.0 mm), the pulp should be extirpated and the root canal dressed with pure calcium hydroxide (e.g. Calasept®, Scandia Dental) immediately prior to splint removal. In teeth whose apical foramen is greater than 1.0 mm, pulpal revascularization is possible. The patient should, therefore, be monitored weekly during the 1st month after injury in order to detect early signs of pulpal infection and inflammatory resorption.

Replantation of avulsed teeth is illustrated in Figs. 8.6 to 8.8 for different trauma situations.

120

### Fig. 8.6. Replantation of a tooth with completed root formation

Replantation of an avulsed maxillary right central incisor in a 19-year-old man. Radiographic examination shows no sign of fracture or contusion of the alveolar socket. The tooth was retrieved immediately after injury and kept moist in the oral cavity. Upon admission to the emergency service, the avulsed incisor was placed in physiologic saline.

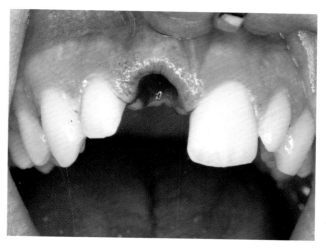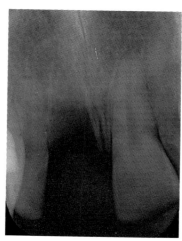

### Rinsing the tooth

The tooth is examined for fractures, position of the level of periodontal attachment and signs of contamination. The tooth is then rinsed with a stream of saline until all visible signs of contamination have been removed. If this is not effective, dirt is carefully removed using a gauze sponge soaked in saline. The coagulum in the alveolar socket is flushed out using a stream of saline.

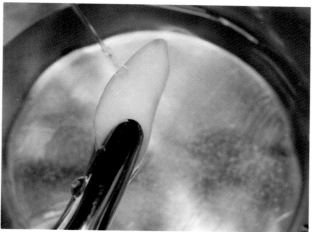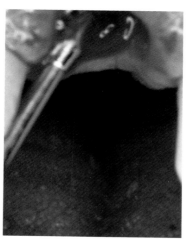

### Replanting the tooth

The tooth is grasped by the crown with forceps and partially replanted in its socket. Replantation is completed using gentle finger pressure. If any resistance is met, the tooth should be removed, placed again in saline and the socket inspected. A straight elevator is then inserted in the socket and an index finger is placed labially. Using lateral pressure, counterbalanced by the finger pressure, the socket wall is repositioned. Replantation can then proceed as described.

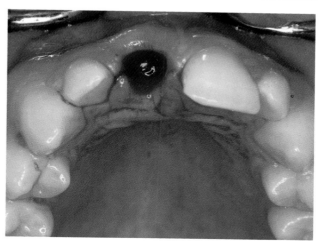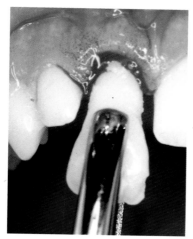

### Splinting

An acid-etch retained splint is applied using the technique described on p. 91. As soon after injury as possible, antibiotic therapy should be instituted. Suggested dosage: penicillin 1 million IU immediately, thereafter 2-4 million IU daily for 4 days.

Good oral hygiene is absolutely necessary in the healing period. This includes brushing with a soft tooth brush and chlorhexidine mouth rinse.

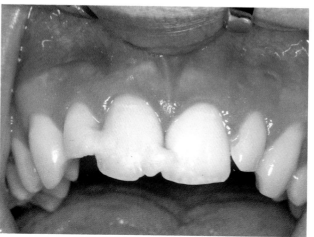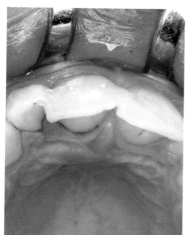

121

### Follow-up: endodontic treatment

One week after replantation, the pulp is extirpated prophylactically to avoid external root resorption. A rubber dam is applied by punching 3 overlapping holes in the dam. The dam is held in place by wedging an extra piece of rubber or dental floss between the last splinted tooth and the adjacent non-splinted tooth in the arch.

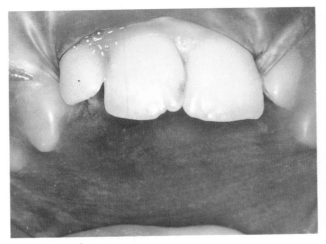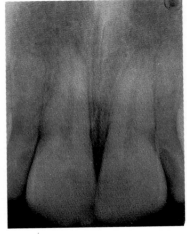

### Extirpating the pulp

After disinfecting the crown of the replanted tooth and crown, an access cavity is prepared to the root canal, its direction following the long axis of the root, to allow sufficient mechanical preparation of the entire canal. The pulp is extirpated by introducing a barbed broach into the midportion of the root canal. A leucocyte zone formed 1-2 mm from the apical foramen will determine the correct amputation level.

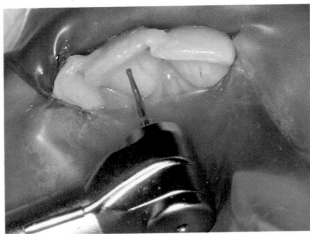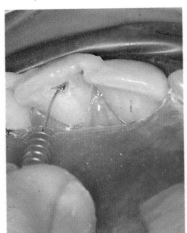

### Amputation level

The coronal pulp chamber is cleansed of pulpal remnants using a small excavator. Careful instruction to the patient as to when he or she just feels the instrument, will dictate the level of chemomechanical root canal preparation and avoid overinstrumentation and post-operative discomfort. This procedure is not associated with pain and therefore does not require the use of local anesthetic.

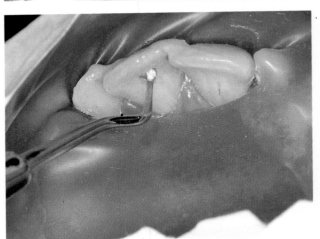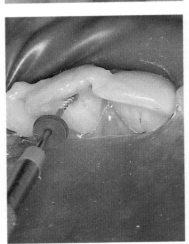

### Preparing the canal

The root canal is prepared with reamers and files using standard endodontic procedures. During this procedure, the root canal is cleansed using sodium hypochlorite as an irrigating medium.

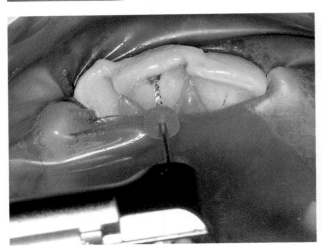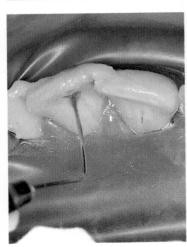

### Placing the calcium hydroxide dressing

After preparation of the root canal, it is flushed with saline. Filling of the root canal with calcium hydroxide paste is facilitated if done in a moist canal. This allows placement of the paste up to the root apex without entrapment of air which could interfere with complete canal obturation. Commercially prepared paste (e.g. Calasept®, Scandia Dental) is injected into the canal and distributed with a lentulo spiral.

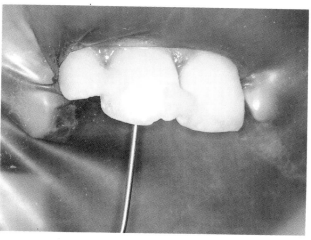

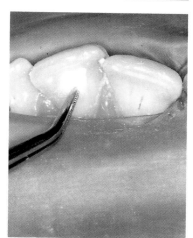

### Condensing the calcium hydroxide dressing

The paste is condensed slightly with paper points. Filling and condensing is repeated 3 times, whereafter a small cotton pellet is placed into the pulp chamber and compressed apically.

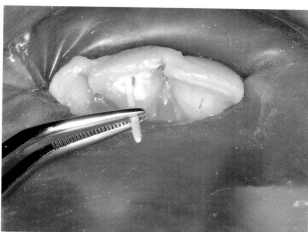

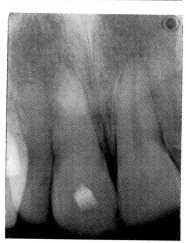

### Closing the access cavity

After removing calcium hydroxide residue from the cavity margins with a water spray, the cavity is air-dried and closed (e.g. IRM®, Cavit®, or glass ionomer cement) to prevent microleakage. Radiographically, calcium hydroxide dressing has the same radiodensity as dentin. The dressing is replaced 1 month later. The root canal can then be obturated with gutta percha and sealer 6-12 months later, when an apical barrier has been formed.

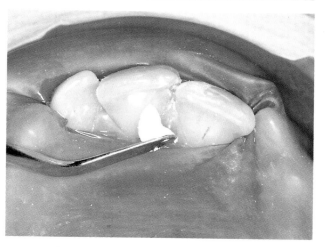

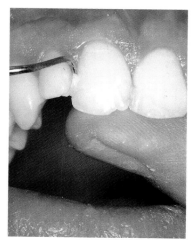

### Splint removal

Once the initial endodontic therapy has been completed, the splinting material can be removed using a fissure bur. The splint is thinned out along its entire span, avoiding gross reduction at any single tooth. The remaining shell of resin interproximally can be removed with a scaler while supporting the replanted tooth incisally. The facial enamel surfaces can be polished with pumice at a later date.

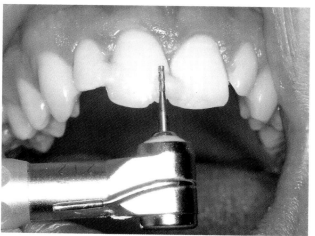

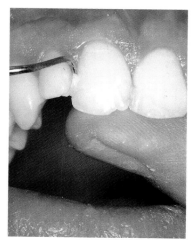

123

## Fig. 8.7. **Replanting a tooth with incomplete root formation**

This 8-year-old boy has avulsed his maxillary left central incisor. The extraalveolar period was 80 min (5 min dry storage; 45 min in saliva; 30 min in physiologic saline). Due to the very patent apical foramen, revascularization of the pulp is considered possible.

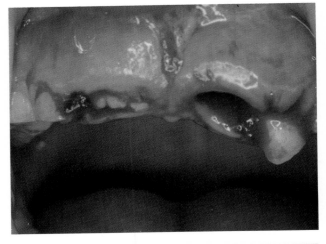 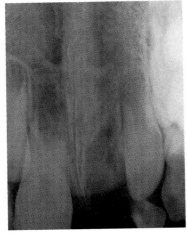

### Rinsing the root surface
The tooth is rinsed carefully with a stream of saline from a syringe. Special care is taken to rinse the apical part of the pulp as well.

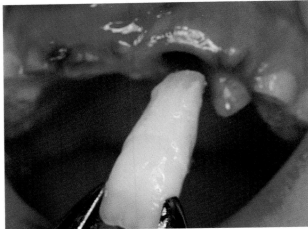 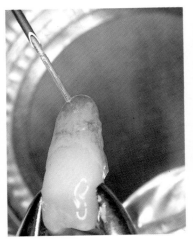

### Replanting the tooth
After cleansing the socket with physiologic saline, the tooth is replanted using the procedure described in the previous case.

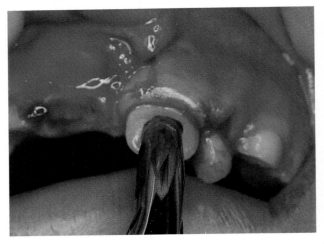 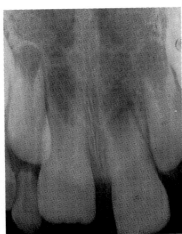

### Monitoring healing
Clinical findings and the radiographic control of healing performed 3 weeks after replantation reveal an infected pulp necrosis.

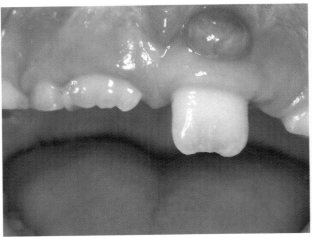 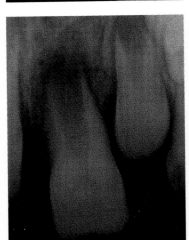

124

## Fig. 8.8. Replanting a tooth with an avital periodontal ligament

In this 21-year-old man, the tooth has been kept dry for 24 hours. Total and irreversible damage to the PDL and pulp can be expected. Furthermore, there is severe contusion of the alveolar socket. In this situation, delayed replantation (to allow healing of the socket), treatment of the root surface (to make it resistant to ankylosis) and endodontic therapy (to prevent inflammatory resorption) is the treatment of choice.

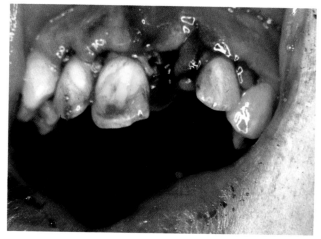 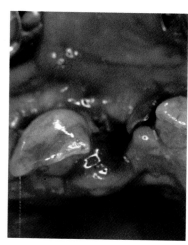

### Treatment of the root surface

The avulsed tooth was in this case kept dry in a refrigerator until healing of the contused socket has taken place. Prior to sodium fluoride treatment, the root surface is rinsed and scraped clean of the dead PDL and the pulp extirpated. The goal of therapy is to incorporate fluoride ions into the dentin and cementum in order to protract the resorption process.

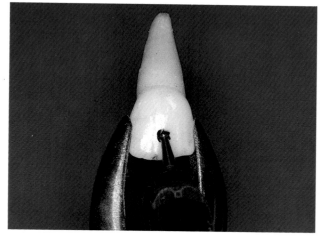 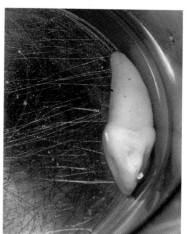

### Fluoride treatment of cementum and dentin

The pulp is extirpated and the root canal enlarged to provide access to the fluoride solution along the entire root canal. The tooth is then placed in a 2.4% solution of sodium fluoride (acidulated to pH = 5.5) for 20 min.

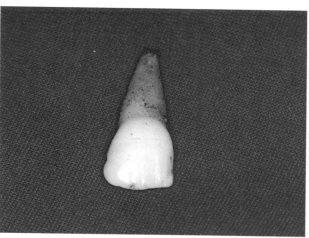 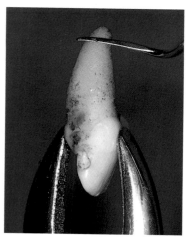

### Endodontic treatment

After rinsing in saline, the root canal is obturated with gutta percha and a sealer.

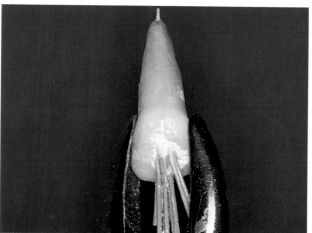 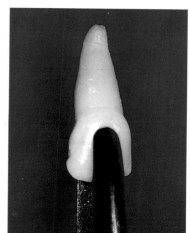

125

**Condition of the socket**
After 3 weeks, the socket area and the contused gingiva are healed.

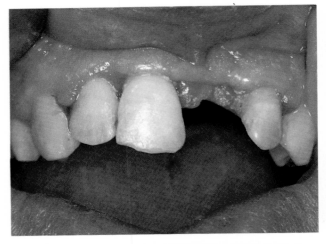 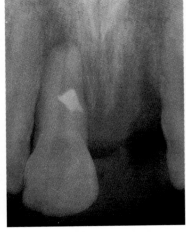

**Replanting the tooth**
The socket is evacuated with excavators and a surgical bur. The tooth is replanted after cleansing with saline to remove excess fluoride solution.

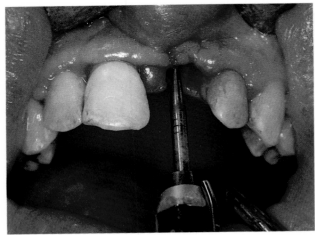 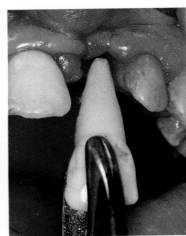

**Splinting**
The tooth is splinted for 6 weeks in order to create a solid ankylosis. In these cases, where no periodontal ligament exists, ankylosis is the only possible healing modality.

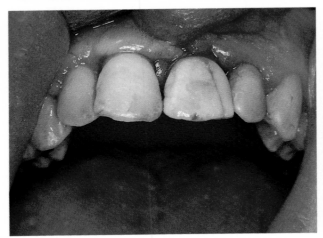 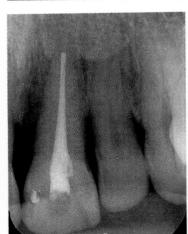

**Follow-up**
Radiographic follow-up over a 3-year period shows no progression of the ankylosis process.

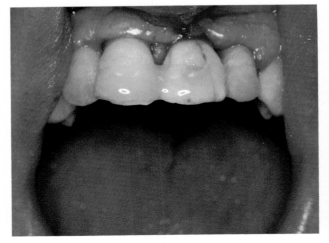 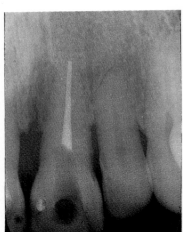

## Follow-up procedures

Replanted teeth should be monitored at regular intervals based upon stage of root development and those times where healing complications might be diagnosed (see Appendix 4, page 161). Thus, a radiographic examination 3 weeks after replantation will permit diagnosis of inflammatory resorption and periapical radiolucency, both indications of infected pulp necrosis (Fig. 8.9). If the radiographic findings vaguely suggest these events, further examinations at 1-week intervals should be made (i.e. for the 1st month). Otherwise, follow-up again at 6 weeks, 3 months and 6 months after injury. A high percussion tone and diminished mobility will reveal ankylosis earlier than radiographs. However, by 6 to 8 weeks, ankylosis can sometimes be seen radiographically (Fig. 8.10).

Immediate endodontic therapy with pulpal extirpation and calcium hydroxide root canal dressing will arrest inflammatory root resorption.

Fig. 8.9. **Development of inflammatory root resorption and pulp necrosis**
Development of external inflammatory root resorption and periapical radiolucency subsequent to replantation. Periapical radiolucency is evident 1 week after replantation and inflammatory root resorption can be detected after 2 weeks.

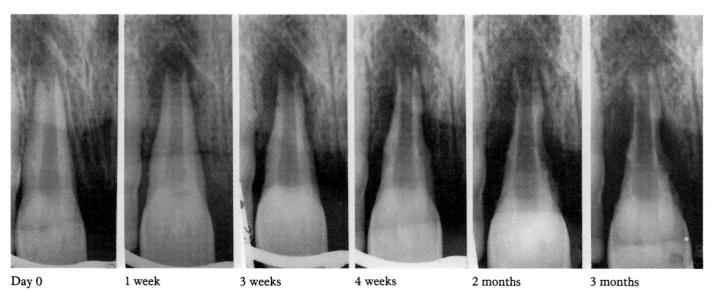

Day 0      1 week      3 weeks      4 weeks      2 months      3 months

127

Fig. 8.10. **Development of ankylosis**
After avulsion in a 25-year-old man, ankylosis could be diagnosed 10 weeks after injury by the percussion test; whereas radiographic diagnosis could be made after 4 months (arrow). Note the slow progression of the resorption process.

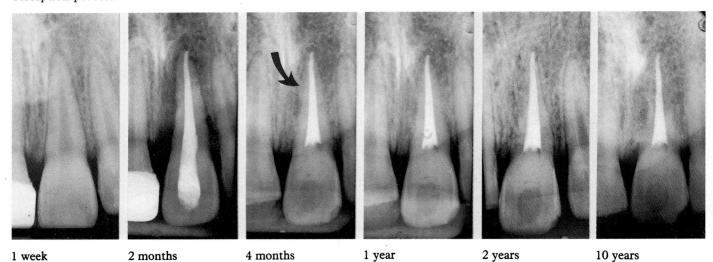

| 1 week | 2 months | 4 months | 1 year | 2 years | 10 years |

## General prognosis

The general outcome of replantation of avulsed teeth is shown in graphs related to pulpal and periodontal ligament healing (Figs. 8.11 and 8.12). However, it should be noted that there is a great variation in healing as related to the time and dry extraalveolar storage (Figs. 8.13 and 8.14).

128

Fig. 8.11. **Pulpal healing after replantation** (after Andreasen et al., 1989)

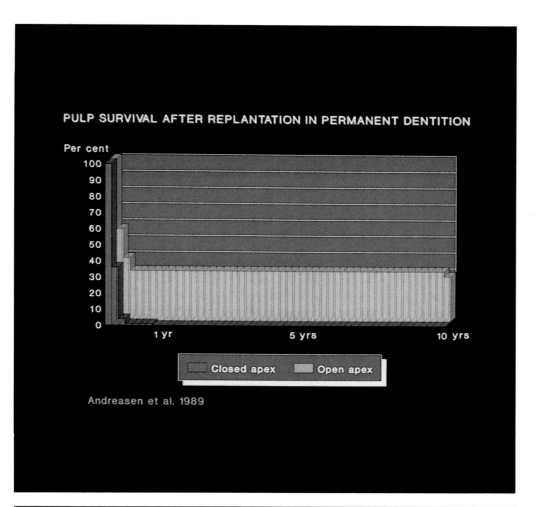

Fig. 8.12. **Periodontal healing after replantation** (after Andreasen et al., 1989)

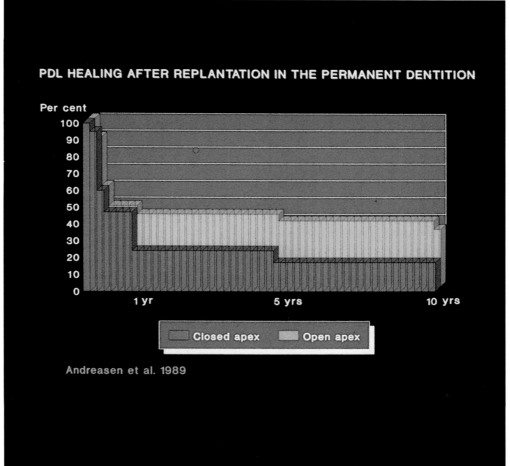

AVULSION INJURIES

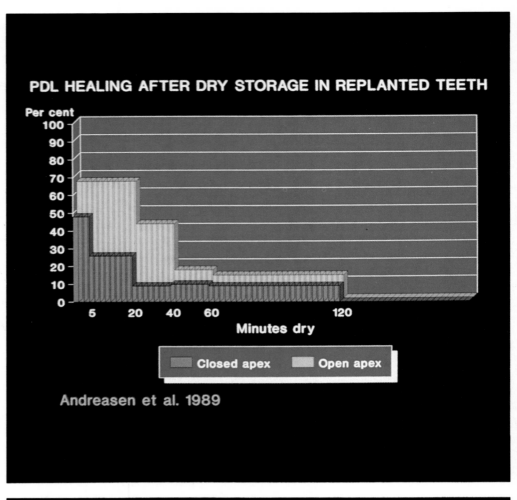

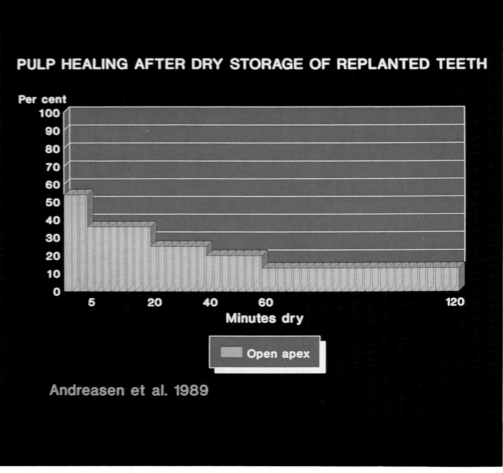

130

## Essentials

- Replantation of avulsed teeth can result in successful healing if there has been only minimal damage to the pulp and periodontal ligament.
- The type of extraalveolar storage and length of storage period have an overwhelming effect upon later healing.
- Replantation should be attempted only if the following conditions can be fulfilled:
  - Absence of gross caries and no major loss of periodontal support prior to injury;
  - Physiological storage of the tooth (in the case of an avital PDL, see below).

### Replantation procedure

- Place the avulsed tooth in saline;
- Examine the socket area;
- Rinse the periodontal ligament and apical foramen with saline;
- Flush the socket with saline;
- Replant the tooth with gentle finger pressure;
- Splint the tooth for 1 week with a semi-rigid splint;
- Begin antibiotic therapy as soon as possible after injury (e.g. penicillin, 1 million IU immediately, thereafter 2-4 million IU four times daily for 4 days);
- If the patient is not covered for tetanus, tetanus vaccine should be administered.

### Follow-up procedures

- In case of a incomplete root formation (i.e. diameter of the apical foramen exceeding 1 mm), pulpal revascularization is a possibility.
- In the case of complete root formation, extirpate the pulp at the same appointment as splint removal (i.e. just prior to removal of the splint) and dress the root canal with calcium hydroxide.
- In case of an *avital PDL* (e.g. extraalveolar dry period longer than 1 hour), resorption-preventing treatment is indicated:
- Remove the PDL and pulp;
- Place the tooth in 2.4% sodium fluoride solution (acidulated to pH = 5.5) for 20 min.;
- Obturate the root canal with gutta percha and a sealer;
- Replant the tooth;
- Splint for 6 weeks.

### Prognosis

Primarily dependent upon extraalveolar period and storage medium. Pulp survival almost nil in teeth with completed root formation and infrequent in teeth with immature root formation. Periodontal ligament healing infrequent and dependent upon the above-mentioned factors.

# Fracture of the alveolar process

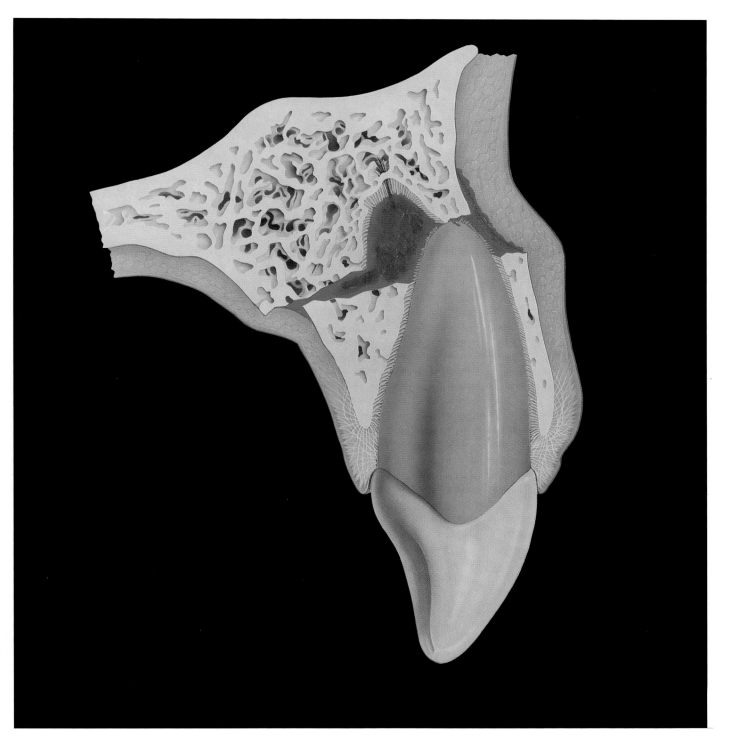

133

Fig. 9.1. **Fracture of the alveolar process**
Both the PDL and the neurovascular supply to the pulp are severed.

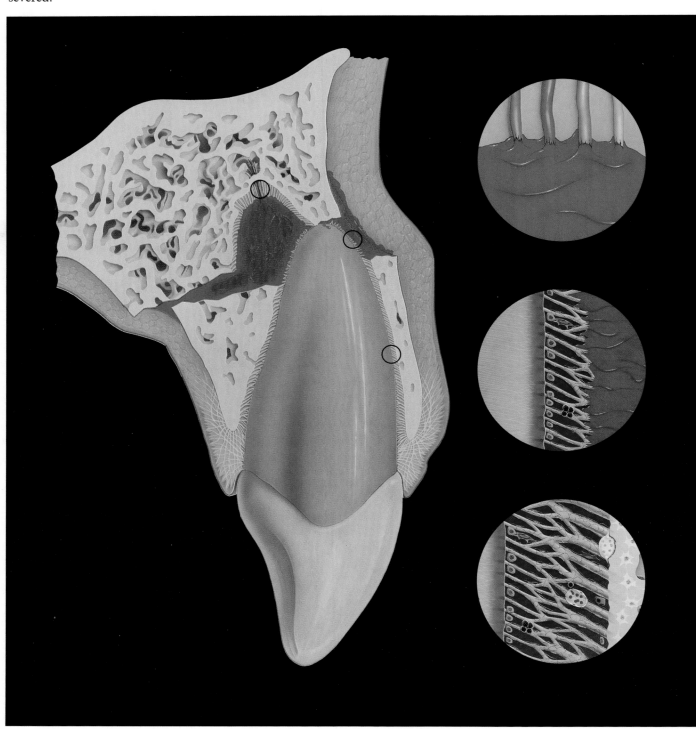

# Pattern of injury and diagnosis

Fracture of the alveolar process is in this context limited to a fracture encompassing the entire alveolar process (Fig. 9.1). Partial alveolar fracture, such as fracture of the labial or lingual bone plate are typical sequelae to lateral luxation and therefore described in that chapter.

Alveolar fracture is a result of a heavy impact to the anterior region. Because of the delicate bone structure of the mandibular incisor region, alveolar fractures are often seen in this region. The fracture usually involves 2 or more teeth and generally follows the PDL of an involved tooth in its vertical course. The horizontal component of the fracture can be seen either at the base of the alveolar process free of the apices, at the level of, or coronal to, the apices.

**Radiographic demonstration** of the entire fracture, including the horizontal and vertical components, is often difficult. Differential diagnosis includes possible root fracture. Thus, multiple radiographs using varying vertical angulations will reveal a fracture line that can move up and down along the root surface in case of an alveolar fracture versus a fracture that remains at the same level of the root in the case of a root fracture.

In this regard, the clinical examination is often more precise in revealing the nature and extent of injury. Thus, when the mobility of one tooth is tested, several teeth move. Also, a hematoma in the adjacent attached gingiva or mucosa is often an indication of alveolar fracture.

## Treatment

**Treatment principles** for fractures of the alveolar process are identical to those for bone fractures in general and consist of repositioning and splinting for 3 – 4 weeks. With respect to repositioning, the problems involved here are similar to those seen following lateral luxation. That is, the root apices are often locked into the facial aspect of the labial bone plate and thus must be

135

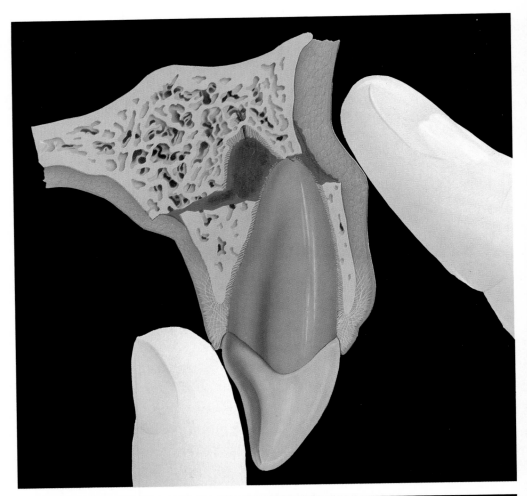

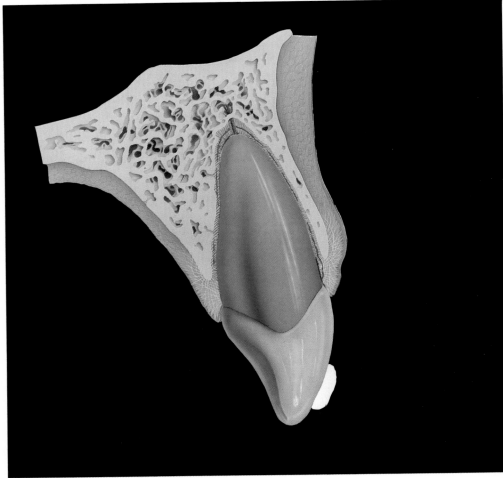

CHAPTER 9

**Fig. 9.3. Fracture of the maxillary alveolar process**
This 21-year-old man suffered a fracture of the maxillary alveolar process from the canine region to the midline.

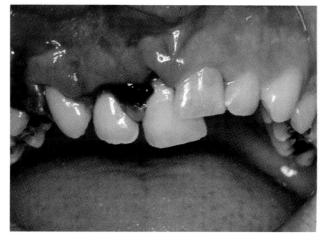 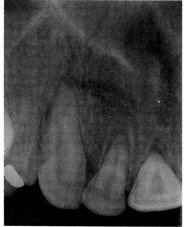

**Anesthetizing the traumatized region**
An infraorbital block and infiltration to the incisive canal are necessary prior to repositioning

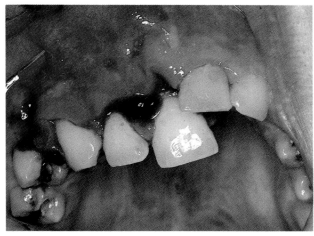 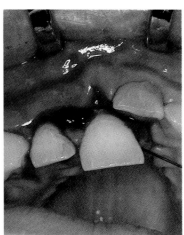

**Repositioning**
With hard finger pressure to the apical region the apices are disengaged. If this is not sufficient then the fragment has to be moved with forceps in a coronal and palatal direction.

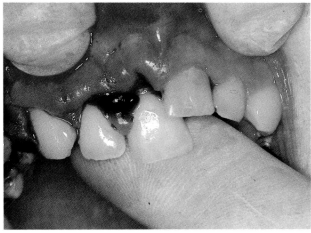 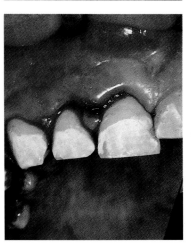

**Splinting**
During curing of the temporary crown and bridge material the patient occludes in order to ensure correct position of the fragment.

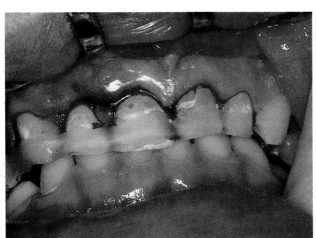 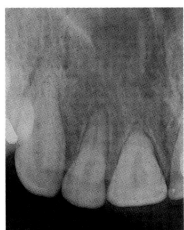

137

FRACTURE OF THE ALVEOLAR PROCESS

further displaced incisally before the tooth and bone segment can be repositioned (Fig. 9.2).

The critical feature in healing of alveolar fractures is pulp related trauma. When the fracture level is apical to the root tips, the vascular supply to the pulp is relatively safe and pulp necrosis rare. In contrast, if the root apices are directly involved in the line of fracture, pulpal healing is jeopardized.

In Fig. 9.3 and 9.4 two examples of repositioning and splinting of alveolar fractures are presented.

**Fig. 9.4. Fracture of the mandibular alveolar process**
An alveolar fracture involving 4 incisors following collision with the steering wheel by a 25-year-old man during an automobile accident.

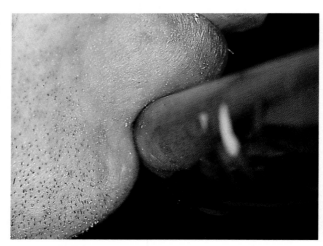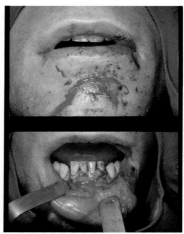

**Apical lock of the fragment**
Attempts at repositioning prove unsuccessful because the apices are locked over the labial bone plate.

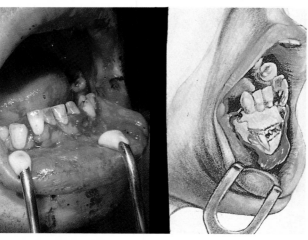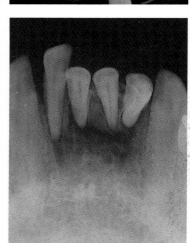

**Disengagement of the apices**
The alveolar fragment is pressed lingually, thereby freeing the apices. Once the apices have been freed, the fragment can be repositioned and the apices will enter their respective sockets.

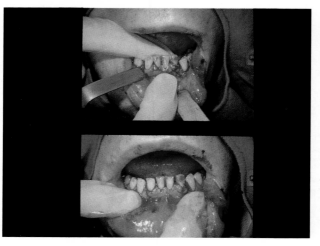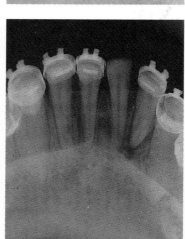

138

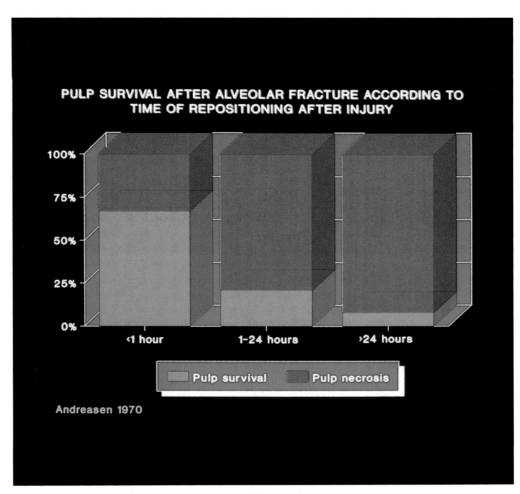

Fig. 9.5. Pulpal healing after alveolar fracture (after Andreasen 1970)

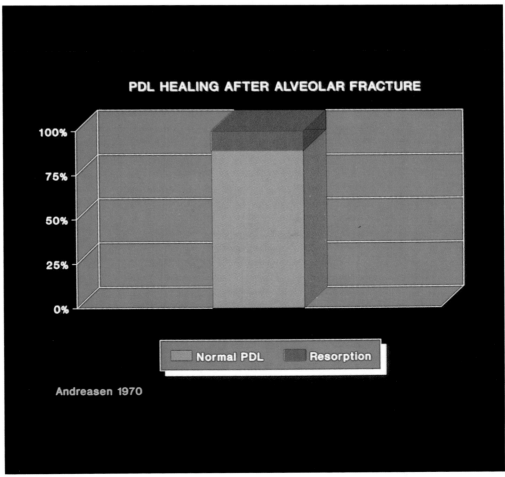

Fig. 9.6. Periodontal healing after alveolar fracture (after Andreasen 1970)

139

## General prognosis

Very few studies have been performed to ascertain healing after alveolar fractures. To date, the only factor related to pulpal healing has been early repositioning of the fracture (Fig. 9.5). Periodontal healing is usually uneventful (Fig. 9.6).

## Essentials

- Verify the extent and position of the fracture clinically and radiographically, using a multiple radiographic exposure technique.
- Place local anesthetic infiltration. Determine whether there is an "apical lock", implying that the fragment cannot be completely repositioned.
- In case of an apical lock, the fragment must first be slightly extruded to free the apices. It is then possible to reposition the fragment.
- Splint the fragment for 3 – 4 weeks, according to the age of the patient.
- Monitor pulpal healing of the involved teeth.

**Prognosis**

The only predictor for pulp necrosis is late repositioning of the fracture. Root resorption is rare.

# Injuries to the primary dentition

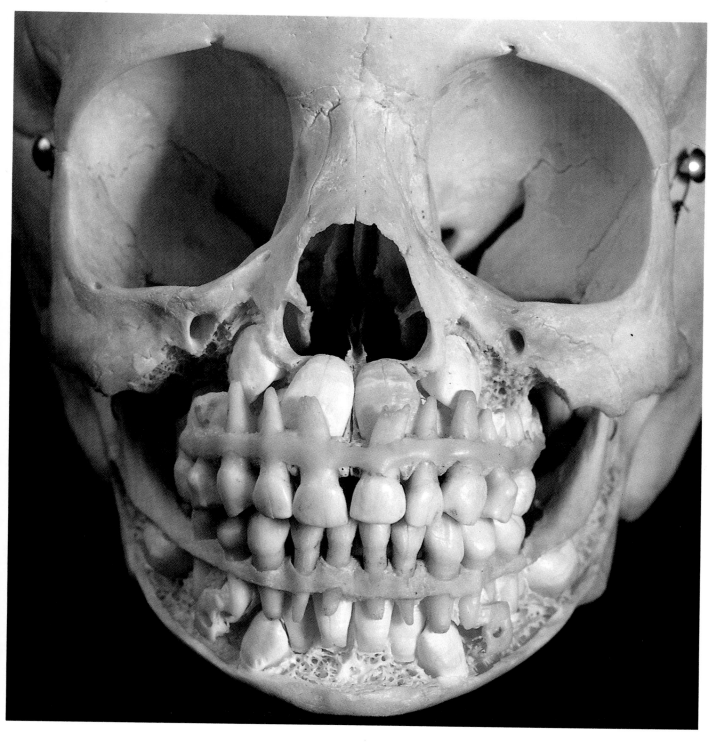

141

Fig. 10.1. **Anatomic relationship between the two dentitions**
The maxilla in a skull of a 3-year-old child. The intimate relation is shown between the primary central incisor and the permanent successor.

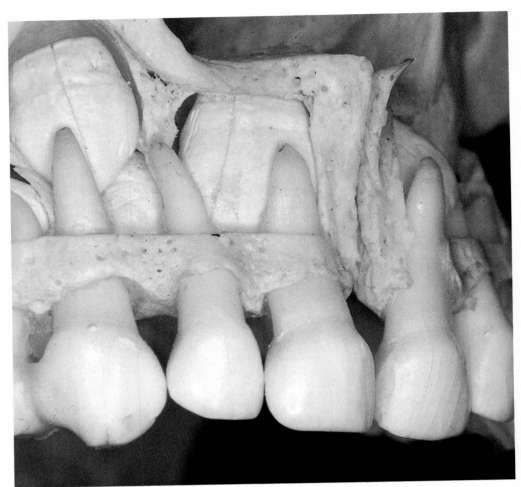

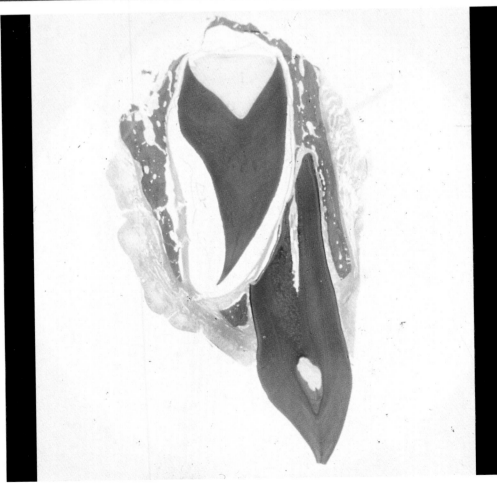

CHAPTER 10

# Pattern of injury and diagnosis

Injuries to the primary dentition are common. Because of the resilient bone surrounding the primary teeth, injuries usually comprise tooth luxations. The close proximity of the two dentitions represents a risk to the permanent dentition in that energy from the acute impact can easily be transmitted to the developing tooth germ (Figs. 10.1 and 10.2). Infection developing subsequent to a primary tooth injury represents another threat to the developing permanent dentition.

The treatment strategy after injury in the primary dentition is, therefore, dictated by concern for the safety of the permanent dentition. To ensure this, the following treatment demands must be respected.

- To ascertain whether or not the displaced primary incisor has invaded the follicle of the developing permanent tooth germ.

If this has occurred, the primary tooth must be removed.

- To monitor healing in the trauma zone so that secondary damage to the developing permanent tooth can be avoided.

**Fig. 10.2. Trauma-related interference with odontogenesis**
An intruded primary tooth may be forced into the follicle and disturb the reduced enamel epithelium and secretory ameloblasts, resulting in enamel discoloration and/or hypoplasia.

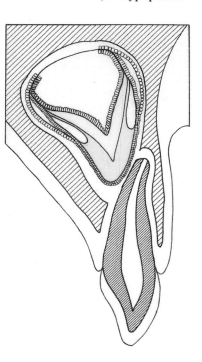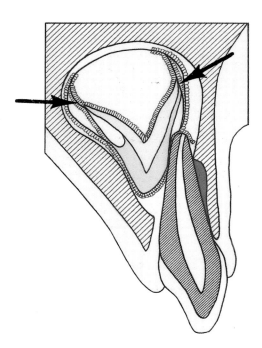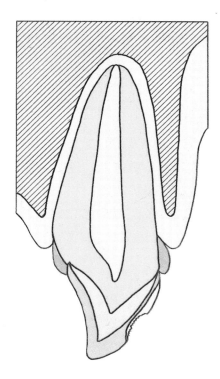

143

**Fig. 10.3. A parent or other adult can assist in stabilizing the child during the radiographic examination**
The parent and child are furnished with lead aprons. One arm is used to hold the child while the other holds the filmholder and stabilizes the child's head against the parent's chest.

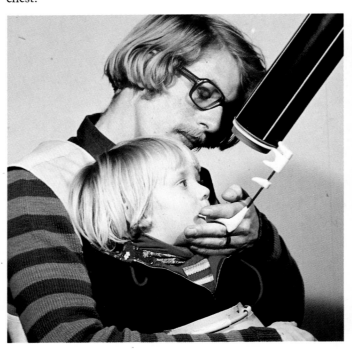

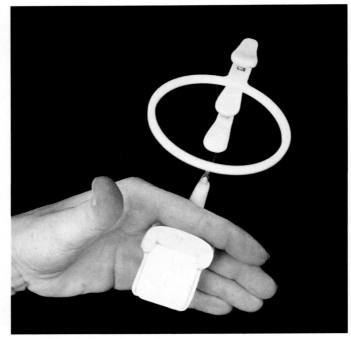

**Fig. 10.4. Schematic illustration of the geometric relationship between an intruded primary incisor and the developing tooth germ and the resultant radiographic image**

If the primary tooth is intruded AWAY from the developing tooth germ, the radiographic image will be FORESHORTENED. If the primary tooth is intruded INTO the developing tooth germ, the radiographic image will be ELONGATED.

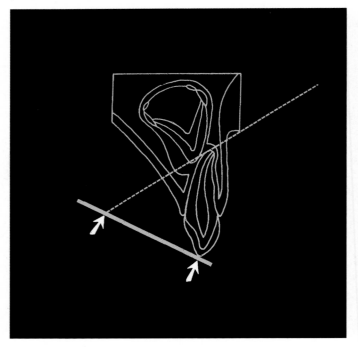

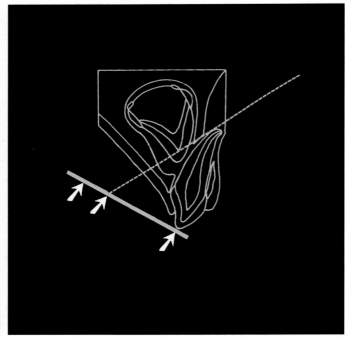

144

CHAPTER 10

Examination of the traumatized primary dentition consists of a clinical examination as well as a radiographic examination of the traumatized region (see Chapter 1). In the case of small and/or unruly children, adult assistance can be necessary (Fig. 10.3). Radiographic examination is also facilitated if it is possible to adjust kilovoltage on the x-ray unit. Thus, for each 10 kVp increase, exposure time can be reduced by one-half without great sacrifice in quality.

With respect to the first treatment demand, this can only be fulfilled by adequate radiographic technique. Two factors are significant: the radiographic dimension of the intruded incisor and the symmetrical orientation of the permanent tooth germs. Regarding the radiographic dimension of the intruded incisor, it can be seen that an incisor which has invaded the follicle of the permanent tooth germ moves away from the x-ray source and thereby becomes *elongated*. In contrast, a primary incisor which is intruded facially, (i.e. away from the permanent follicle and towards the x-ray source) becomes *foreshortened* (Fig. 10.4).

Fig. 10.5. **Radiographic demonstration of displacement of the developing permanent tooth germ following intrusion of the primary incisor**
The distance between the incisal edge and mineralization front of the involved developing tooth germ is shorter than the same distance in the non-involved tooth germ, implying luxation of the involved tooth germ. Although the displaced primary tooth was removed, a slight dilaceration of the permanent crown developed.

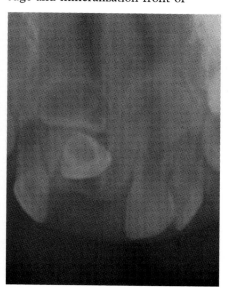
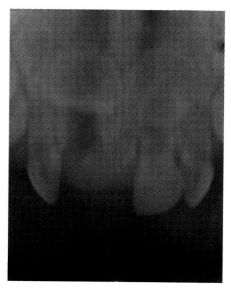
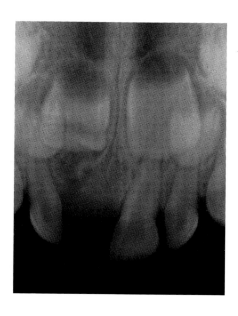

Until crown formation is complete and root formation begins, it is possible that intrusion of a primary incisor can lead to luxation of the permanent tooth germ. Unless diagnosed and treated immediately, tooth germ luxation can lead to severe malformation of the crown of the affected permanent tooth. Diagnostic features of tooth germ luxation are the following. If the intruded primary incisor has invaded the follicle of the permanent tooth germ and thereby displaced it, the distance between its incisal edge and the mineralization front will be shorter than the same distance of its counterpart (Fig. 10.5). However, for diagnosis to be valid, the radiograph must be symmetrical with respect to midline alignment. For further illustration of these concepts, see later under treatment of intrusions.

## Treatment

### Crown fractures
Most fractures consist of chipped enamel or superficial enamel-dentin fractures. In both situations, slight grinding of sharp edges is sufficient. In cases of pulp exposure, a pulpotomy can be performed if the child is cooperative. Otherwise, extraction is often the treatment of choice.

### Crown-root fractures
In these cases, the pulp is usually involved and extraction is almost always the treatment of choice.

Fig. 10.6. **Root fracture with associated healing complication**
These root fractures occurred at the age of 4 years. Due to severe displacement, both coronal fragments were extracted. The root tips remained in situ and were resorbed normally.

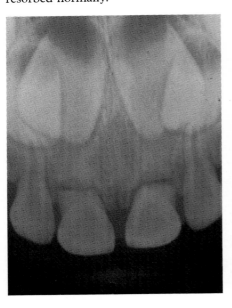
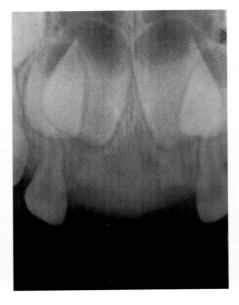
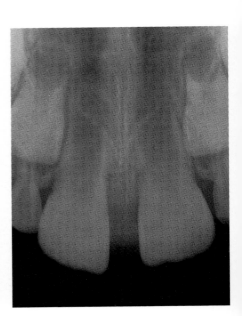

### Root fractures

These cases can be treated conservatively. Splinting is usually difficult or impossible to perform in the primary dentition (due to diminutive tooth size and lack of patient cooperation). Healing must, therefore, occur despite mobility at the fracture line, usually resulting in interposition of connective tissue. In some instances, infection will occur in the coronal pulp, in which case it is important to consider that only the coronal fragment need be extracted and that the apical fragment can be left to resorb physiologically (Fig. 10.6).

### Lateral luxation

Lateral luxation of primary teeth is the most common injury; and usually does not require treatment, as the crown is displaced lingually and the apex and cortical bone plate labially, i.e. away from the developing tooth germ. Unless occlusion dictates otherwise, a laterally luxated incisor can be left untreated. Over a period of 1-2 months, tongue pressure will reposition the tooth (Fig. 10.7).

In rare instances (e.g. after a fall with an object in the mouth), the laterally luxated tooth will be displaced in the opposite direction, i.e. with the apex forced into the follicle. In this case, extraction is the treatment of choice in order to prevent further damage to the permanent tooth germ.

Fig. 10.7. **Lateral luxation, repositioning indicated**
This 2-year-old boy suffered a lateral luxation. Due to occlusal interference, the tooth had to be repositioned. At a subsequent control, there is evidence of pulpal revascularization, as the root canal has become obliterated.

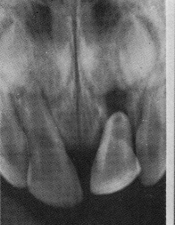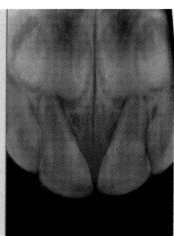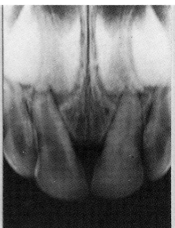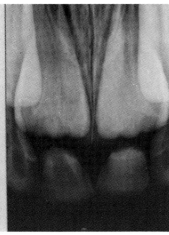

147

## Intrusion

Due to the labial tilt of primary incisor roots, most roots of intruded primary incisors will be forced through the labial bone plate as a result of an axial impact. Foreshortening of the intruded incisor in an occlusal radiographic exposure normally confirms this direction of displacement (Fig. 10.8). In such case, reeruption of the primary incisor should be anticipated and will normally occur within 2-4 months after injury (Fig. 10.9).

In the few cases where intrusive forces displace the primary incisor root into the follicle zone, removal of the displaced tooth is essential to relieve the pressure upon the odontogenic tissue within the follicle (Fig. 10.10).

When displacement of the primary incisor requires removal, it is essential that the extraction procedure does not elicit further injury to the developing permanent successor (Fig. 10.10). Therefore, it is necessary that certain guidelines are followed. Thus, because of the eminent risk of collision with the permanent tooth germ, elevators should never be used to luxate the primary inci-

**Fig. 10.8. Intrusion, the follicle not invaded**
This 4-year-old boy suffered intrusion of a central incisor. A lateral radiograph demonstrated no interference with the follicle. At later examination, reeruption of the intruded incisor is seen. There is no sign of pulp necrosis.

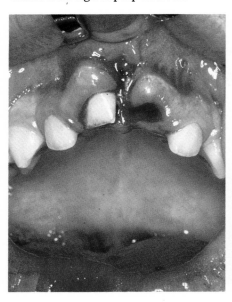 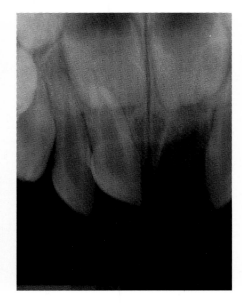 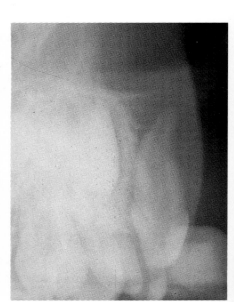

CHAPTER 10

**Fig. 10.9. Spontaneous re-eruption of an intruded primary incisor**
This 2-year old boy suffered an intrusion of the right central incisor. The foreshortened appearance of the intruded tooth implies labial displacement. Spontaneous re-eruption is therefore anticipated.

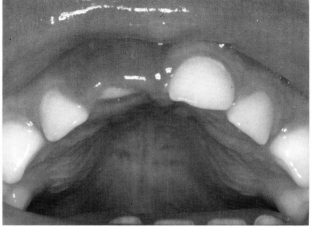 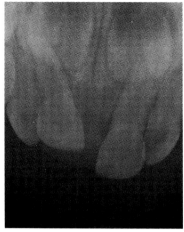

**Follow-up, 2 months after injury**
The tooth has erupted approximately 2 mm coronally.

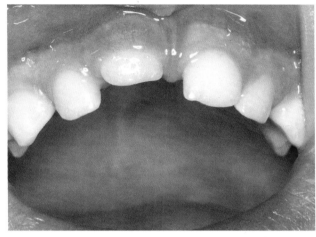 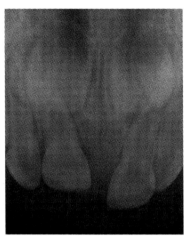

**Follow-up, 3 months after injury**
The tooth lacks 1 mm for complete eruption.

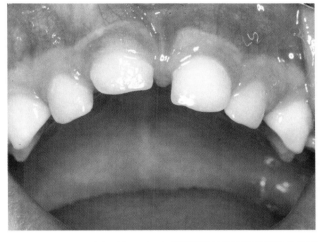 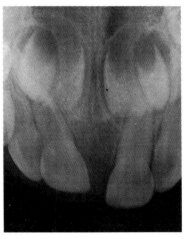

**Follow-up, 1 year after injury**
The tooth is in normal position. Crown color is normal and the radiographs show no sign of pathology.

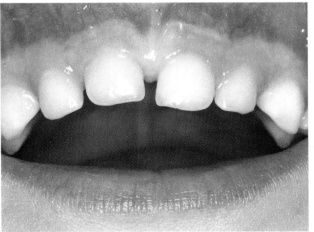 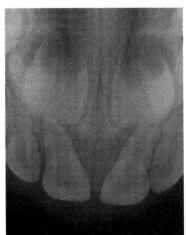

INJURIES TO THE PRIMARY DENTITION

**Fig. 10.10. Intrusion, severe follicle invasion**

This 1-year-old boy received an axial impact, resulting in complete intrusion of the central incisor. Note the displacement of the permanent tooth germ in the follicle. Removal of the primary incisor is mandatory.

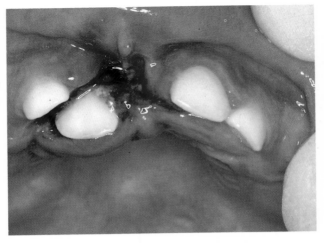 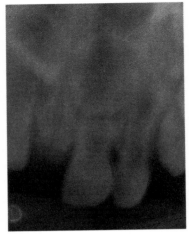

**Removing the displaced tooth**

Using sedation and topical anesthesia, the tooth is grasped proximally with forceps and removed in a labial direction. The fractured and displaced palatal bone is repositioned with digital pressure and a suture placed to close the entrance to the socket.

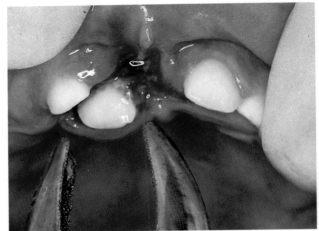 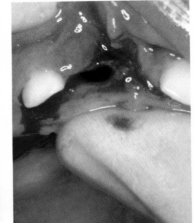

**Follow-up**

At examination 1 week later, a slight change in the position of the tooth germ is seen.

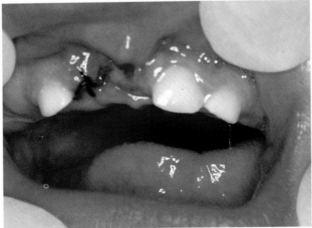 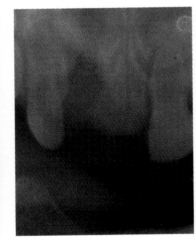

**Disturbance in eruption**

At the age of 6 years, it is evident that a crown dilaceration has developed.

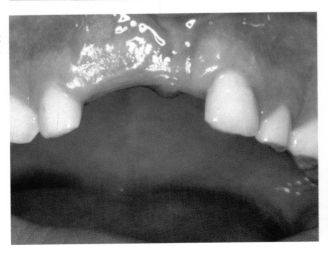 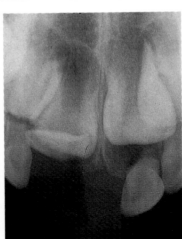

sor. Forceps should be the only instrument employed for this purpose. Moreover, the primary incisor should be grasped by the proximal surfaces, as there is a risk that if the tooth is grasped faciolingually that the forceps could glide along the crown apically into the follicle zone. Once grasped mesiodistally, the displaced incisor should be lifted out of its socket in a labial and axial direction. Finally, once extracted, digital pressure should be applied to the buccal and lingual aspects of the socket to reposition the displaced bone plates. If necessary, a single suture should be used to approximate the facial and oral gingiva and thereby narrow the entrance to the socket.

In those cases where extraction is not indicated, one must be aware of the risk of infection due to impaction of bacterial plaque at the site of trauma. Signs of infection include swelling, spontaneous bleeding, abscess formation and fever. In these cases, the traumatized incisor must be removed and antibiotic therapy instituted (Fig. 10.11).

**Fig. 10.11. Acute infection after intrusion**
This 3-year-old boy suffered intruson of the 2 central incisors. As the root tips were displaced away from the developed tooth germ, spontaneous eruption was anticipated.

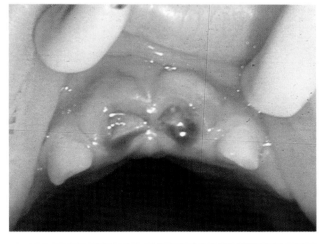 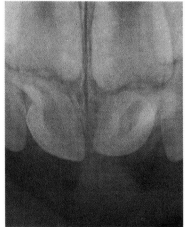

**Follow-up, 2 weeks after injury**
Acute infection with swelling and pus formation around the displaced incisors has developed.

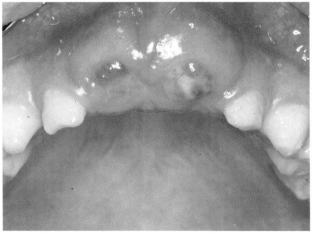 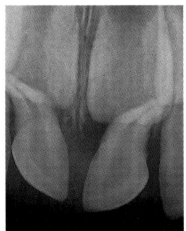

151

## Avulsion

Replantation of avulsed primary teeth is contraindicated, as pulp necrosis is such a frequent event. Moreover, there is a risk of further injury to the permanent tooth germ by the replantation procedure whereby the coagulum can be forced into the area of the follicle.

**10.12. Clinical and radiographic follow-up**
Reversal of coronal discoloration of a subluxated primary incisor.

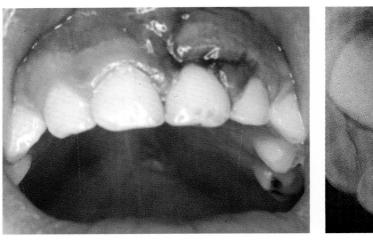

**Follow-up, 3 weeks after injury**
Intense reddish brown discoloration is seen.

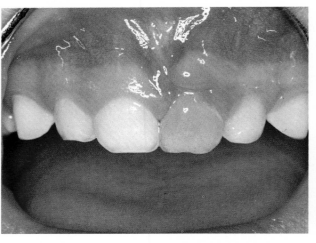
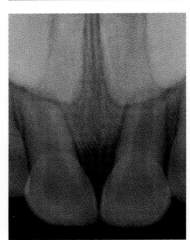

**Follow-up, 1 year after injury**
The color has changed to yellow and the radiographs demonstrate pulp canal obliteration.

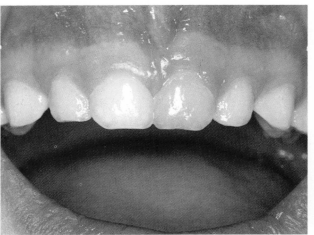
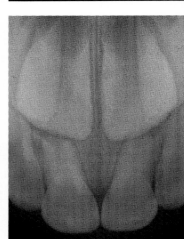

## Follow-up procedures

All traumas in the primary dentition resulting in displacement of the primary teeth (i.e. implying possible damage to the neurovascular supply) should be monitored, as infected pulp necrosis is a likely event, affecting approximately half of all displaced teeth. A suggested follow-up schedule includes radiographic and clinical examination 1 and 2 months after injury (to ascertain spontaneous reeruption of the displaced tooth and early pulpal complications); and 1 year (to diagnose late pulpal complications as well as eventual malformation of the permanent successor).

With respect to pulp necrosis, it should be considered that reversible color changes of the crown are very frequent (Fig. 10.12).

## General prognosis

Data on the prognosis of traumatized primary teeth are scarce with respect to the risk of trauma to the developing permanent tooth germ. However, both age at time of injury and type of luxation appear to influence the permanent dentition (Figs. 10.13 and 10.14).

Fig. 10.13. **Risk of developmental disturbances in the permanent dentition according to the type of trauma** (after Andreasen & Ravn, 1970)

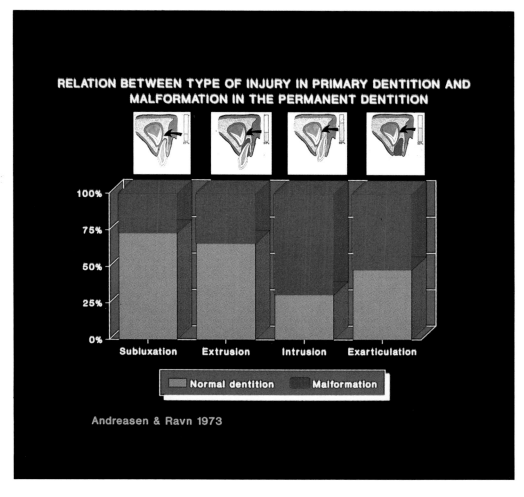

RELATION BETWEEN TYPE OF INJURY IN PRIMARY DENTITION AND MALFORMATION IN THE PERMANENT DENTITION

Subluxation  Extrusion  Intrusion  Exarticulation

Normal dentition  Malformation

Andreasen & Ravn 1973

153

Fig. 10.14. **Risk of developmental disturbances in the permanent dentition according to the age of patient** (after Andreasen & Ravn, 1970)

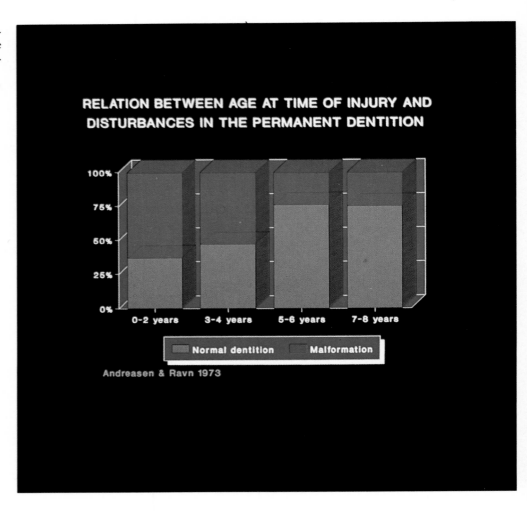

RELATION BETWEEN AGE AT TIME OF INJURY AND
DISTURBANCES IN THE PERMANENT DENTITION

Andreasen & Ravn 1973

## Essentials

– Verify eventual collision between a displaced primary tooth and its permanent successor.
– If this has occurred, remove the displaced incisor.
– Otherwise, the displaced position of the luxated incisor can be accepted (unless it interferes with occlusal function); and spontaneous repositioning can be expected. With the conservative approach to dental trauma, one must be aware of the possible risk of infection due to impaction of bacterial plaque at the trauma site. In this case, the luxated incisor must also be removed.
– Monitor healing regularly with routine clinical and radiographic examinations (i.e. after 1 and 2 years).

# Appendix 1

Emergency record for acute dental trauma

| Patient's name | |
| Birthdate | |

| Date of examination: | Referred by: |
| Time of examination: | Referring diagnosis: |

| | |
|---|---|
| *General medical history:* any serious illness? <br> *If yes,* explain. | yes no |
| *Previous dental injuries?* <br> *If yes,* <br>    When? <br>    Which teeth were injured? <br>    Treatment given and by whom? | yes no |
| *Present dental injury:* <br>    Date:          Time: <br>    Where? <br>    How? | |
| Have you had or have now *headache?* | yes no |
| Have you had or have now *nausea?* | yes no |
| Have you had or have now *vomiting?* | yes no |
| Were you *unconscious* at the time of injury? <br> *If yes,* for how long (minutes)? | yes no |
| Can you *remember* what happened before, during or after the accident? | yes no |

The emergency record is constructed so that wherever a question is answered by *yes,* more details must be provided. Finally, the last question in the record is whether the examiner has re-read the chart. This is a reminder to check that all relevant points have been registered.

155

**Emergency record for acute dental trauma**

---

Is there pain from *cold air?*  | yes | no
If yes, *which teeth?*

---

Is there pain or tenderness from *occlusion?*  | yes | no
If yes, *which teeth?*

---

*Constant pain?*  | yes | no
If yes, *which teeth?*

---

*Treatment elsewhere?*  | yes | no
If yes, *what treatment?*

---

After *exarticulation,* the following information is needed:
*Where* were the teeth found (dirt, asphalt, floor, etc.)?
*When* were the teeth found?
Were the teeth *dirty?*
How were the teeth *stored?*
Were the teeth *rinsed* and *with what* prior to replantation?
*When* were the teeth replanted?
Was *tetanus antitoxoid* given?
Were *antibiotics* given?
   *Antibiotic?*
   *Dosage?*

---

**Objective examination**
Is the patient's general condition affected?  | yes | no
If yes, *pulse*
      *blood pressure*
      *pupillary reflex*
      *cerebral condition*
Objective findings beyond the head and neck?  | yes | no
If yes, *type* and *location*
Objective findings within the head and neck?  | yes | no
If yes, *type* and *location*

156

**Emergency record for acute dental trauma**

**Objective examination – Extraoral findings (contd.)**

| | | |
|---|---|---|
| Bleeding from nose, or rhinitis | yes | no |
| Bleeding from ext. auditory canal | yes | no |
| Double vision or limited eye movement | yes | no |
| Palpable signs of fracture of facial skeleton | yes | no |
| If yes, *location of fracture* | | |

**Objective examination – Intraoral findings**

| | | |
|---|---|---|
| Lesions of the *oral mucosa* | yes | no |
| If yes, *type* and *location* | | |
| *Gingival lesion* | yes | no |
| If yes, *type* and *location* | | |
| *Tooth fracture* | yes | no |
| If yes, *type* and *location* | | |
| *Alveolar fracture* | yes | no |
| If yes, *type* and *location* | | |

Supplemental information:

**General condition of the dentition**

| | | | |
|---|---|---|---|
| Caries | poor | fair | good |
| Periodontal status | poor | fair | good |
| Horizontal occlusal relationship | undr bite | over jet | norm |
| Vertical occlusal relationship | deep | open | norm |

**Radiographic findings**

Tooth dislocation

Root fracture

Bone fracture

Pulp canal obliteration

Root resorption

**Photographic registration**  yes  no

157

APPENDIX 1

**Emergency record for acute dental trauma**

Diagnoses (check appropriate boxes and designate tooth no. or indicate correct anatomical region)

| | |
|---|---|
| ☐ Infraction | ☐ Skin abrasion |
| ☐ Complicated crown fracture | ☐ Skin laceration |
| ☐ Uncomplicated crown fracture | ☐ Skin contusion |
| ☐ Complicated crown-root fracture | ☐ Mucosal abrasion |
| ☐ Uncomplicated crown-root fracture | ☐ Mucosal laceration |
| | ☐ Mucosal contusion |
| ☐ Root Fracture | |
| ☐ Alveolar fracture | ☐ Gingival abrasion |
| ☐ Mandibular fracture | ☐ Gingival laceration |
| ☐ Maxillary fracture | ☐ Gingival contusion |
| ☐ Concussion | *Supplementary remarks:* |
| ☐ Subluxation | |
| ☐ Extrusion | |
| ☐ Lateral luxation | |
| ☐ Intrusion | |
| ☐ Exarticulation | |

**Treatment plan**
*At time of injury:*                                           *Final therapy:*
Repositioning (time finished)
Fixation (time finished)
Pulpal therapy (time finished)
Dentinal coverage (time finished)

*Chart re-*read by examining dentist                    ☐ yes    ☐ no

158

# Appendix 2

**Clinical examination form for the time of injury and follow-up examinations**

| | Tooth no. | 12 | | 11 | | 21 | | 22 | |
|---|---|---|---|---|---|---|---|---|---|
| **T I M E** | Date | | | | | | | | |
| | Tooth color<br>  normal<br>  yellow<br>  red<br>  grey<br>  crown restoration | | | | | | | | |
| **O F** **I N J U R Y** | Displacement (mm)<br>  intruded<br>  extruded<br>  protruded<br>  retruded | | | | | | | | |
| | Loosening (0-3) | | | | | | | | |
| | Tenderness to percussion ( + / − ) | | | | | | | | |
| | Pulp test (value) | | | | | | | | |
| | Ankylosis tone ( + / − ) | | | | | | | | |
| | Occlusal contact ( + / − ) | | | | | | | | |
| **C O N T R O L** | Fistula ( + / − ) | | | | | | | | |
| | Gingivitis ( + / − ) | | | | | | | | |
| | Gingival retraction (mm) | | | | | | | | |
| | Abnormal pocketing ( + / − ) | | | | | | | | |

Each column represents an examination of a given tooth. The first column for each tooth gives the values from the time of injury. *Only* the parameters listed in the top half of the form ("Time of injury") are to be recorded at the time of injury. The information from this examination as well as the information collected on the emergency record are used to determine the final diagnoses for the injured teeth. Those parameters *and* the last four (fistula, gingivitis, gingival retraction, abnormal pocketing) are to be registered at all follow-up controls.

159

# Appendix 3

**Clinical and radiographic findings with the various luxation types**

| Findings | Concussion | Subluxation | Extrusion | Lateral Luxation | Intrusion |
|---|---|---|---|---|---|
| **Clinical** | | | | | |
| Abnormal mobility | − | + | + | −(+) | −(+) |
| Tenderness to percussion | + | +(−)* | +/− | −(+) | −(+) |
| Percussion sound** | normal | dull | dull | metallic | metallic |
| Response to pulp testing | +/− | +/− | −(+) | −(+) | −(+) |
| Clinical dislocation | − | − | + | + | + |
| Radiographic dislocation | − | − | + | + | + |

  * A sign in parentheses indicates a finding of rare occurrence.
** Teeth with incomplete root formation and teeth with marginal or periapical inflammatory
    lesions will also elicit a dull percussion sound.

# Appendix 4

Summary of treatment and follow-up procedures and recall schedule following the various trauma types

| Post-traumatic interval* | Radiographic exposure for various trauma types | | |
| --- | --- | --- | --- |
| | Luxation of 21** | Replantation of 21 | Root fracture of 21 |
| Time of injury | OI 11,21*** BI 12,11,21,22 | OI 11,21 BI 12,11,21,22 | OI 11,21 BI 12,11,21,22 |
| 1 week | | BI 21,22£$ | |
| 2-3 weeks | OI 11,21£$ | BI 21,22 | OI 11,21 |
| 6-8 weeks | BI 12,11,21,22£ | BI 12,11,21,22 | BI 12,11,21,22 |
| 3 months | | BI 21,22 | BI 12,11,21,22£ |
| 6 months | | BI 21,22 | |
| 1 year | BI 12,11,21,22 | BI 12,11,21,22 | BI 12,11,21,22 |
| 2, 3, 4 years | | BI 21,22 | |
| 5, 10, 15 years | BI 12,11,21,22 | BI 12,11,21,22 | BI 12,11,21,22 |

  * All examinations include radiographs as well as information from the clinical examination form (see Appendix 2).

  ** Tooth designation is according to the FDI two-digit system.

  *** Regarding radiographic exposure, OI implies "Occlusal Identical", or occlusal exposures; BI implies "bisecting identical". Both designations imply the use of standardized techniques and filmholder.

£ Removal of fixation. The following fixation periods are suggested. The reader is referred to the respective chapters for details: Replantation, 1 week; Extrusion, 2-3 weeks; Lateral luxation, 3-8 weeks (depending on radiographic findings); Intrusion, see text for discussion of repositioning and fixation; Root fracture, 3 months.

$ Begin endodontic therapy: Replantation, after 1 week, Intrusion, after 2 weeks.

# Bibliography

## Chapter 1. Examination of the patient

1. ANDREASEN FM, ANDREASEN JO. Diagnosis of luxation injuries. The importance of standardized clinical, radiographic and photographic techniques in clinical investigations. *Endod Dent Traumatol* 1985; 1: 160–9.
2. ANDREASEN JO. *Traumatic injuries of the teeth,* 2nd Ed. Copenhagen: Munksgaard International Publishers, 1981.
3. ANDREASEN JO. Etiology and pathogenesis of traumatic dental injuries. A clinical study of 1,289 cases. *Scand J Dent Res* 1970; 78: 329–42.
4. ANDREASEN JO, RAVN JJ. Epidemiology of traumatic dental injuries to primary and permanent teeth in a Danish population sample. *Int J Oral Surg* 1972; 1: 235–9.
5. *Application of the International Classification of Diseases and Stomatology.* IDC-DA. Geneva: World Health Organization, 1966.
6. KOPEL HM, JOHNSON R. Examination and neurologic assessment of children with oro-facial trauma. *Endod Dent Traumatol* 1985; 1: 155–159.
7. OIKARINEN K. Pathogenesis and mechanism of traumatic injuries to teeth. *Endod Dent Traumatol* 1987; 3: 220–223.
8. RAVN JJ. Dental injuries in Copenhagen schoolchildren, school years 1967-1972. *Comm Dent Oral Epidemiol* 1974; 2: 231–45.

## Chapter 2. Crown fracture

1. ANDREASEN FM, RINDUM JL, MUNKSGAARD EC, ANDREASEN JO. Bonding of enamel-dentin crown fractures with GLUMA® and resin. *Endod Dent Traumatol* 1986; 2: 277–80.
2. ANDREASEN FM, ANDREASEN JO. Prognosis of crown fractures with and without periodontal injury. 1989: In preparation.
3. BRÄNNSTRÖM M. Observations on exposed dentine and the corresponding pulp tissue. A preliminary study with replica and routine histology. *Odont Revy* 1962: 13: 235–45.
4. CVEK M. A clinical report on partial pulpotomy and capping with calcium hydroxide in permanent incisors with complicated crown fracture. *J Endod* 1978; 4: 232–7.
5. CVEK M, LUNDBERG M. Histological appearance of pulps after exposure by a crown fracture, partial pulpotomy, and clinical diagnosis of healing. *J Endod* 1983; 9: 8–11.
6. FUKS AB, CHOSACK A, KLEIN H, EIDELMAN E. Partial pulpotomy as a treatment alternative for exposed pulps in crown-fractured permanent incisors. *Endod Dent Traumatol* 1987; 3: 100–2.

7. GOLDBERG F, MASSONE EJ, SPIELBERG C. Evaluation of the dentinal bridge after pulpotomy and calcium hydroxide dressing. *J Endod* 1984; 10: 318–20.
8. HALLET GEM, PORTEOUS JR. Fractured incisors treated by vital pulpotomy. A report on 100 consecutive cases. *Br Dent J* 1963; 115: 279–87.
9. HELLE A, SIRKKANEN R, EVALAHTI M. Repair of fractured incisal edges with UV-light polymerized and self-polymerizing fissure sealants and composite resins. Two year report of 93 cases. *Proc Finn Dent Soc* 1975; 71: 87–90.
10. HOLLAND R, DE SOUZA, V, DE MELLO W, NERY MJ, BERNABE PFE, FILHO JAO. Permeability of the hard tissue bridge formed after pulpotomy with calcium hydroxide: a histologic study. *J Am Dent Assoc* 1979; 99: 472–5.
11. KOCH G, PAULANDER J. Klinisk uppföljning av compositrestaureringar utförda med emaljetsningsmetodik. *Swed Dent J* 1976; 69: 191–6.
12. LIM KC, KIRK EEJ. Direct pulp capping: a review. *Endod Dent Traumatol* 1987; 3: 213–9.
13. MADER C. Restoration of a fractured anterior tooth. *J Am Dent Assoc* 1978; 96: 113–5.
14. OLGART L, BRÄNNSTRÖM M, JOHNSON G. Invasion of bacteria into dentinal tubules. Experiments in vivo and in vitro. *Acta Odontol Scand* 1974; 32: 61–70.
15. RAVN JJ. Follow-up study of permanent incisors with enamel cracks as a result of an acute trauma. *Scand J Dent Res* 1981; 89: 117–23.
16. RAVN JJ. Follow-up study of permanent incisors with enamel fractures as a result of an acute trauma. *Scand J Dent Res* 1981; 89: 213–7.
17. RAVN JJ. Follow-up study of permanent incisors with enamel-dentin fractures after acute trauma. *Scand J Dent Res* 1981; 89: 355–65.
18. RAVN JJ. Follow-up study of permanent incisors with complicated crown fractures after acute trauma. *Scand J Dent Res* 1982; 90: 363–72.
19. SMALES RJ. Incisal angle adhesive restorations: a two-year clinical survey of three materials. *Australian Dent J* 1977; 22: 267–71.
20. SIMONSEN RJ. Restoration of a fractured central incisor using original tooth fragment. *J Am Dent Assoc* 1982; 105: 648–50.
21. TZIAFAS D, BELTES P. Pulp capping with calcium hydroxide: diagnostic value of radiographic findings. *Endod Dent Traumatol* 1988; 4: 260–4.
22. QVIST V, STRÖM C, THYLSTRUP A. Two-year assessment of anterior resin restorations inserted with two acid-etch restorative procedures. *Scand J Dent Res* 1985; 93: 343–50.

**163**

## Chapter 3. Crown-root fracture

1. BESSERMANN M. Ny behandlingsmetode af kronerodfrakturer. *Tandlægebladet* 1978; 82: 441–4.
2. HEITHERSAY GS. Combined endodontic-orthodontic treatment of transverse root fractures in the region of the alveolar crest. *Oral Surg* 1973; 36: 404–15.
3. INGBER JS. Forced eruption: Part II. A method of treatment nonrestorable teeth – periodontal and restorative considerations. *J Periodont* 1976; 47: 203–16.
4. KAHNBERG K-E. Surgical extrusion of root-fractured teeth – a follow-up study of two surgical methods. *Endod Dent Traumatol* 1988; 4: 85–89.
5. PERSSON M, SERNEKE D. Ortodontisk framdragning av tand med cervikal rotfraktur for att möjliggöra kronersättning. *Tandläkartid* 1977; 69: 1263–9.
6. TEGSJÖ U, VALERIUS-OLSSON H, OLGART K. Intra-alveolar transplantation of teeth with cervical root fractures. *Swed Dent J* 1978; 2: 73–82.

## Chapter 4. root fracture

1. ANDREASEN JO, HJØRTING-HANSEN E. Intraalveolar root fractures: radiographic and histologic study of 50 cases. *J Oral Surg* 1967; 25: 414–26.
2. ANDREASEN FM, ANDREASEN JO, BAYER T. Prognosis of root fractured permanent incisors – prediction of healing modalities. *Endod Dent Traumatol* 1989; 5: 11–22.
3. ANDREASEN FM, ANDREASEN JO. Resorption and mineralization processes following root fracture of permanent incisors. *Endod Dent Traumatol* 1988; 4: 202–14.
4. CVEK M. Treatment of non-vital permanent incisors with calcium hydroxide. IV. Periodontal healing and closure of the root canal in the coronal fragment of teeth with intra-alveolar fracture and vital apical fragment. *Odont Revy* 1974; 25: 239–45.
5. JACOBSEN I, ZACHRISSON BU. Repair characteristics of root fractures in permanent anterior teeth. *Scand J Dent Res* 1975; 83: 355–64.
6. JACOBSEN I. Root fractures in permanent anterior teeth with incomplete root formation. *Scand J Dent Res* 1976; 84: 210–7.
7. ZACHRISSON BU, JACOBSEN I. Long-term prognosis of 66 permanent anterior teeth with root fracture. *Scand J Dent Res* 1975; 83: 345–54.
8. RAVN JJ. En klinisk og radiologisk undersøgelse af 55 rodfrakturer i unge permanente incisiver. *Tandlægebladet* 1976; 80: 391–6.

## Chapter 5. Concussion and subluxation

1. ANDREASEN FM, VESTERGAARD PEDERSEN B. Prognosis of luxated permanent teeth – the development of pulp necrosis. *Endod Dent Traumatol* 1985; 1: 207–20.
2. ANDREASEN FM. Pulpal healing after luxation injuries and root fracture in the permanent dentition. *Endod Dent Traumatol* 1989; 5: 111–31.
3. EKLUND G, STÅLHANE I, HEDEGÅRD B. Traumatized permanent teeth in children aged 7–15 years. III. A multivariate analysis of posttraumatic complications of subluxated and luxated teeth. *Swed Dent J* 1976; 69: 179–89.

BIBLIOGRAPHY

4. ROCK WP, GORDON PH, FRIEND LA, GRUNDY MC. The relationship between trauma and pulp death in incisor teeth. *Br Dent J* 1974; 136: 236–9.
5. STÅLHANE I, HEDEGÅRD B. Traumatized permanent teeth in children aged 7–15 years. Part II. *Swed Dent J* 1975; 68: 157–69.

## Chapter 6. Extrusion and lateral luxation

1. ANDREASEN JO. Luxation of permanent teeth due to trauma. A clinical and radiographic follow-up study of 189 injured teeth. Scand *Scand J Dent Res* 1970; 78: 273–86.
2. ANDREASEN FM, VESTERGAARD PEDERSEN B. Prognosis of luxated permanent teeth – the development of pulp necrosis. *Endod Dent Traumatol* 1985; 1: 207–20.
3. ANDREASEN FM, YU Z, THOMSEN BL. The relationship between pulpal dimensions and the development of pulp necrosis after luxation injuries in the permanent dentition. *Endod Dent Traumatol* 1986; 2: 90–8.
4. ANDREASEN FM. Transient apical breakdown and its relation to color and sensibility changes. *Endod Dent Traumatol* 1986; 2: 9–19.
5. ANDREASEN FM. Histological and bacteriological study of pulps extirpated after luxation injuries. *Endod Dent Traumatol* 1988; 4: 170–81.
6. ANDREASEN FM, YU Z, THOMSEN BL, ANDERSEN PK. The occurrence of pulp canal obliteration after luxation injuries in the permanent dentition. *Endod Dent Traumatol* 1987; 3: 103–115.
7. ANDREASEN FM. Pulpal healing after luxation injuries and root fracture in the permanent dentition. *Endod Dent Traumatol* 1989; 5: 111–131.
8. DUMSHA T, HOVLAND EJ. Pulpal prognosis following extrusive luxation injuries in permanent teeth with closed apexes. *J Am Dent Assoc* 1982; 36: 410–2.
9. HERFORTH M. *Traumatische Schädigungen der Frontzähne bei Kindern und Jugendlichen im Alter von 7 bis 15 Jahren*. Berlin: Quintessenz Verlags-GmbH. 1982.
10. OIKARINEN K. Functional fixation for traumatically luxated teeth. *Endod Dent Traumatol* 1987; 3: 224–8.
11. OIKARINEN K, GUNDLACH KKH, PFEIFER G. Late complications of luxation injuries to teeth. *Endod Dent Traumatol* 1987; 3: 296–303.
12. ROCK WP, GRUNDY MC. The effect of luxation and subluxation upon the prognosis of traumatized incisor teeth. *J Dent* 1981; 9: 224–30.

## Chapter 7. Intrusion

1. ANDREASEN JO. Luxation of permanent teeth due to trauma. A clinical and radiographic follow-up study of 189 injured teeth. *Scand J Dent Res* 1970; 78: 273–86.
2. ANDREASEN FM, YU Z, THOMSEN BL. The relationship between dimensions and the development of pulp necrosis after luxation injuries in the permanent dentition. *Endod Dent Traumatol* 1986; 2: 90–8.
3. ANDREASEN FM, VESTERGAARD PEDERSEN B. Prognosis of luxation permanent teeth – the development of pulp necrosis. *Endod Dent Traumatol* 1985; 1: 207–20.

## Chapter 8. Avulsion/exarticulation

1. ANDERSSON L, BODIN I, SÖRENSEN S. Progression of root resorption following replantation of human teeth after extended extraoral storage. *Endod Dent Traumatol* 1989; 5: 38–47.
2. ANDREASEN JO, HJØRTING-HANSEN E. Replantation of teeth. I. Radiographic and clinical study of 110 human teeth replanted after accidental loss. *Acta Odontol Scand* 1966; 24: 263–86.
3. ANDREASEN JO, HJØRTING-HANSEN E. Replantation of teeth. II. Histological study of 22 replanted anterior teeth in humans. *Acta Odontol Scand* 1966; 24: 287–306.
4. ANDREASEN JO. Periodontal healing after replantation of traumatically avulsed human teeth. Assessment by mobility testing and radiography. *Acta Odontol Scand* 1975; 33: 325–35.
5. ANDREASEN JO, NYGAARD J, BORUM M, ANDREASEN FM. Replantation of 400 traumatically avulsed permanent incisors. I. Diagnosis of healing complications. In preparation.
6. ANDREASEN JO, NYGAARD J, BORUM M, ANDREASEN FM. Replantation of 400 avulsed permanent incisors. II. Factors related to pulp healing and root growth. In preparation.
7. ANDREASEN JO, NYGAARD J, BORUM M, ANDREASEN FM. Replantation of 400 avulsed permanent incisors. III Factors related to Periodontal ligaenil healing. In preparation.
8. ANDREASEN JO. Atlas of replantation and transplantation of teeth. Fribourg: Mediglobe, 1989 (in press).
9. CVEK M, GRANATH L-E, HOLLENDER L. Treatment of non-vital permanent incisors with calcium hydroxide. III. Variation of occurrence of ankylosis of reimplanted teeth with duration of extra-alveolar period and storage environment. *Odont Revy* 1974; 25: 43–56.
10. HAMMARSTRÖM L, PIERCE A, BLOMLÖF L, FEIGLIN B, LINDSKOG S. Tooth avulsion and replantation – A review. *Endod Dent Traumatol* 1986; 2: 1–8.
11. KLING M, CVEK M, MEJÀRE I. Rate and predictability of pulp revascularization in therapeutically reimplanted permanent incisors. *Endod Dent Traumatol* 1986; 2: 83–89.

microscopic study of 117 injured permanent teeth. *Scand J Dent Res* 1970; 79: 219–83.
4. BASSAT YB, BRIN I, FUKS A, ZILBERMAN Y. Effect of trauma to the primary incisors on permanent successors in different developmental stages. *Pediatric Dentistry* 1985; 7: 37–40.
5. DYNESEN H, RAVN JJ. Rodfrakturer i det primære tandsæt. *Tandlægebladet* 1973; 77: 865–8.
6. LIND V, WALLIN H, EGERMARK-ERIKSSON I, BERNHOLD M. Indirekta traumaskador. Kliniska skador på permanenta incisiver som följd av trauma mot temporära incisiver. *Sv Tandläkforb Tid* 1970; 62: 738–56.
7. RAVN JJ. Sequelae of acute mechanical traumata in the primary dentition. *J Dent Child* 1968; 35: 281–9.
8. RAVN JJ. Developmental disturbances in permanent teeth after exarticulation of their primary predecessors. *Scand J Dent Res* 1975; 83: 131–4.
9. RAVN JJ. Developmental disturbances in permanent teeth after intrusion of their primary predecessors. *Scand J Dent Res* 1976; 84: 137–41.
10. SELLISETH N-E. The significance of traumatised primary incisors on the development and eruption of permanent teeth. *Trans Eur Orthod Soc* 1970; 46: 443–59.
11. ZILBERMAN Y, FUKS A, BASSAT YB, BRIN I, LUSTMANN J. Effect of trauma to primary incisors on root development of their permanent successors. *Pediatric Dentistry* 1986; 4: 289–293.

## Chapter 9. Fractures of the alveolar process

1. ANDREASEN JO. Fractures of the alveolar process of the jaw. A clinical and radiographic follow-up study. *Scand J Dent Res* 1970; 78: 263–72.

## Chapter 10. Injuries to the primary dentition

1. ANDREASEN JO, RAVN JJ. The effect of traumatic injuries to primary teeth on their permanent successors. II. A clinical and radiographic follow-up study of 213 injured teeth. *Scand J Dent Res* 1970; 79: 284–94.
2. ANDREASEN JO, RAVN JJ. Enamel changes in permanent teeth after trauma to their predecessors. *Scand J Dent Res* 1973; 81: 203–9.
3. ANDREASEN JO, SUNDSTRØM B, RAVN JJ. The effect of traumatic injuries to primary teeth on their permanent successors. I. A clinical, radiographic, microradiographic and electron-

**165**

# Index

166